EXERCISES
FOR
CARDIAC
RECOVERY

EXERCISES

FOR

CARDIAC
RECOVERY

The Strong Heart
Fitness Program for
Life After Heart Attack
& Heart Surgery

WILLIAM SMITH, M.S.

KEITH BURNS, M.S.

AND

CHRISTOPHER VOLGRAF

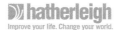
hatherleigh
Improve your life. Change your world.

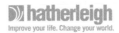
Exercises for Cardiac Recovery
Text copyright © 2018 William Smith, Keith Burns and Christopher Volgraf

Library of Congress Cataloging-in-Publication Data is available upon request.
ISBN: 978-1-57826-706-4

Cover design by Heather Daugherty
Interior Design by Cynthia Dunne

Printed in the United States

10 9 8 7 6 5 4 3 2 1

 Your health starts here! Workouts, nutrition, motivation,
community...everything you need to build a better body
from the inside out!

Visit us at www.getfitnow.com for videos, workouts, nutrition, recipes,
community tips, and more!

Consult your physician before beginning any exercise program. The author and pub-
lisher of this book and workout disclaim any liability, personal or professional, resulting from the misapplication of any of the following procedures described in this
publication.

CONTENTS

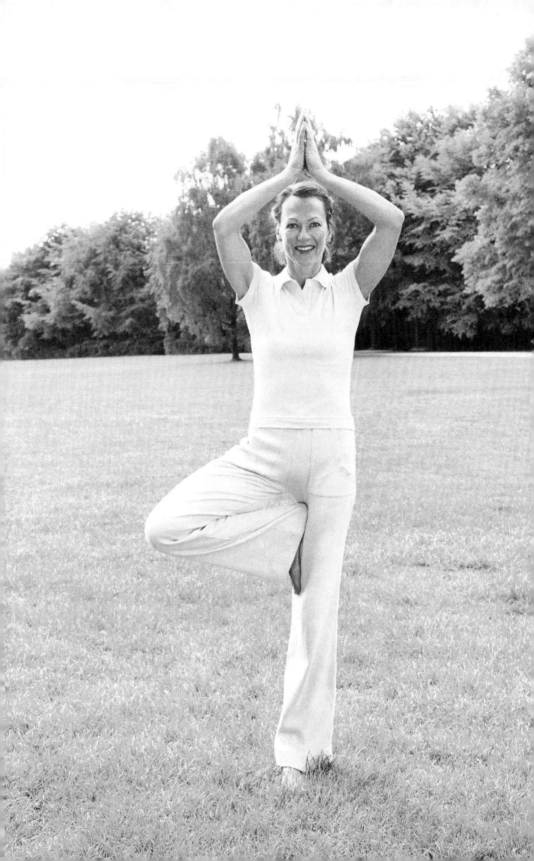

THE STRONG HEART FITNESS PROGRAM

DO YOU...

- have a job where you sit at a desk all day?
- need effective, proven heart-healthy exercising programming?
- struggle to find time in your busy professional life for daily movement?
- spend hours a day commuting with limited time to elevate your heart rate?
- need to start heart-healthy exercise programming after a physician's recommendation?
- recognizing the importance of a healthy lifestyle?
- need a self-monitored routine for risk factor modification?
- want a resource for supporting healthy living initiatives
- need a brief, daily routine addressing full-body strength

Then the Strong Heart Fitness Program is for YOU!

ARE YOU EXPERIENCING...

- fatigue and lethargy from normal, daily activities
- decreased muscle toning and strength
- poor balance and movement quality
- inability to concentrate and focus from inactivity
- headaches and neck discomfort from forward head posture
- poor recovery heart rate after movement
- poor circulation and edema
- inability to perform enjoyable activities such as walking, swimming and related heart-centric movements

Then the Strong Heart Fitness Program is for YOU!

Our society is experiencing the widening effects of inactivity. Approximately 80% of diseases are preventable. This means that even short bouts of movement throughout the day can have dramatic results on your overall health. Small changes and good habits lead to very positive change, and it starts today! Whether you're a busy parent, a caregiver for an elderly parent, a patient cleared to for self-monitored exercise, or an active older adult, we all can make simple changes in our daily lives that have a huge impact.

When I started my medical residency in the late 1970s, it was common for the patient to stay in hospital for up to 6 weeks, and then be told that they should avoid physical activity for another 6 weeks—that was "standard" cardiac recovery. Unfortunately, what we saw as a result were "cardiac cripples," individuals who had lost mental and physical health in addition to losing endurance, muscle mass, and bone mass.

During my now more than 35 years practicing cardiology, cardiac recovery has undergone major changes, but these have been very slow to spread. I eventually became an "intensivist," practicing in the MICU (Medical Intensive Care Unit) and the CCU (Cardiac Care Unit). Although I took care of critical care patients, my primary concern was just keeping them alive and out of the hospital. I was introduced early on to "cardiac rehabilitation" programs, intended for survivors of heart attacks or congestive heart failure, but I would have little participation in their care after they left the CCU.

Later, I became involved with imaging methods that promised to discover "developing" heart disease, long before it caused disabilities. I began working with what was called the "Cardiovascular Health Clinic," where we dealt with teaching individuals about their cardiovascular risk factors (high blood pressure, high cholesterol, inactivity, and the like). One component of the assessment was to perform a symptom-limited treadmill exercise test, looking for heart rhythm issues, hypertension, and possibly exercise-induced abnormalities in heart blood flow. After this was done, I and/or one of my colleagues would sit down with the patient and give them an "exercise prescription."

The patter would go like this: "Exercise on a treadmill or a bicycle, spending 5 minutes gradually building up to your 'target' heart rate (derived from parameters from the prior stress test), spend 20 minutes at a sustained 'target' heart rate, and then 'cool down' for 5 minutes."

The "exercise prescription" called for a total of 30 minutes of treadmill/stationary bicycle, at least 3 times per week…and that was it. No mention of strength training or maintaining flexibility. All the same, I thought this was sound advice from my instructors and continued to prescribe this method to my patients.

As I moved from being a Critical Care Cardiologist to a Cardiac Rehab director, I still pursued my passion of using imaging, specifically Cardiac CT, to define "early" heart disease (rather than dealing with late heart disease in my days of critical care). The pursuit of this passion led me to my current situation, as Director of Cardiac Imaging at the Princeton Longevity Center.

The Princeton Longevity Center was a "new" environment, one which brought me into direct and daily contact with certified Exercise Physiologists working as active members of the Prevention Team. I slowly learned from this association, which included all three authors of *Exercises for Cardiac Recovery*, that what I had been taught as a "one size fits all" post-cardiac recovery plan was too simple an approach, that adaptations of interval training emphasizing both weight/strength training, flexibility, and aerobic conditioning can and should be individualized to the patient.

I became the student again and was taught and mentored by William Smith, Keith Burns, and especially Christopher Volgraf—and I am a better physician and cardiologist because of it.

Exercises for Cardiac Recovery is for the patient, the physician, and the student in exercise physiology. In these pages, the authors lay out how to apply physical activity, no matter how defined, to improve physical abilities, mental/physical strength, and flexibility, to afford you the best physical path to your own cardiac recovery.

—John A. Rumberger, PhD, MD, FACC, FSCCT
   Director of Cardiac Imaging
   The Princeton Longevity Center

INTRODUCTION

In writing this book, we set a goal for ourselves. We want to re-define the common perception of what cardiac recovery can be, working from a fitness-based perspective (after all, that's our specialty).

Once patients leave the hospital or rehabilitation setting, they are typically given a general maintenance program based on acceptable industry standards. This program—by industry standards—may well be excellent, but it comes with a caveat. Because the individual in question is no longer a patient in a controlled, supervised setting, unknown variables are introduced, including the person's level of personal commitment—their level of motivation. Clients who experience a medical "scare" (such as an emergency room visit) may be more motivated to get healthy once cleared by their doctor for exercise.

But what about the majority of the population, those who have controllable risk factors that *can* be modified through lifestyle and behavior changes?

For this reason, self-motivation is vital to maintain any gains made in the hospital setting. Likewise, if you are looking to move from a state of inactivity to one of regular movement, being able to stay committed and moving forward is vital to both achieve and maintain the desired results.

That's where we come in. *Exercises for Cardiac Recovery* offers professional guidance based on best practice, heart healthy guidelines, all while challenging readers to try new, more dynamic approaches to fitness.

CARDIAC RECOVERY FIT TIP: HEART FUNCTION AND PHYSICAL ACTIVITY

We've all heard that physical activity is good for your cardiovascular system—an intricate anatomical system comprised of the heart, blood vessels, diaphragm and related structures. Increasingly strenuous physical activity helps to strengthen the pumping function of the heart and encourages faster recovery after exertion, among many other positive effects.

THE NEW MODEL OF HEALTHCARE

Cardiac health means more than exercising regularly and eating well. Cardiac health is something that is affected by your environment, your social support systems and you're your level of intellectual stimulation.

This is the key to our Strong Heart Fitness approach: the idea that you are a complete being, and that your heart is your life's center, pumping oxygen-rich nutrients to your body regardless of the situation.

This approach is based on the new model for healthcare, which is completely changing how healthcare providers treat their patients and is even starting to trickle down local gyms. Prevention is becoming a larger part of equation (with health educators and fitness professionals taking a bigger role as a result), not only for individuals but for the communities they live in. This broad initiative is called population health, and it represents a radical re-thinking of how health is handled. Local YMCAs are now working with insurance carriers to cover diabetes prevention and treatment programs. In New Jersey, Horizon Blue Cross, an insurance carrier, offers a program called Horizon Be-Fit, which reimburses insured members to the tune of 50 percent of their monthly gym fee just for exercising 12 times a month.

As fitness has become more local and cost effective, fitness professionals have been able to take an even larger role in the preventive equation. This goes hand in hand with the trend of offering increasingly progressive and specialized fitness training—finding a "niche" for every "body." The medical exercise and post-rehabilitation fields are now catering to active baby boomers and seniors that are living longer. Specialty fitness centers such as CrossFit have been found to draw more able-bodied participants who are training for general health or even to maximize participation in challenging events like Tough Mudder.

Outside of the gym, local and community-based heart healthy resources include farmers' markets, co-operative fruit and vegetable gardens, and farm-to-table eating. The recent trend towards urban re-migration is enabling residents to connect with their communities on a local level, enabling greater access to no-cost physical activities and authentically healthy food.

AN INTEGRATIVE SYSTEM OF HEALTHCARE

By working closely with existing healthcare systems, communities are beginning to take back their health through the creation of "integrative systems" of care, which connect acute care (such as you'd receive in a larger hospital setting) with resources in the community. This new model monitors patient welfare even after discharge, as they transition into outpatient or community-based care. Reimbursement models, such as those employed by Medicare (and which private payers tend to imitate) are penalizing health systems for patients being re-admitted for the same or similar conditions. Integrative care is now being recognized as the ideal solution to the problems of efficient health care and increased patient recovery. By connecting patients with resources where they live, work and play, we ensure that they are properly cared for in respect to their heart health needs.

ACSM'S "EXERCISE IS MEDICINE" INITIATIVE

Perhaps the most impactful medical program in the last decade is the American College of Sports Medicine's Exercise is Medicine® initiative. Exercise is Medicine (EIM) is a global health initiative managed by the American College of Sports Medicine (ACSM) that is focused on encouraging primary care physicians and other health care providers to include physical activity when designing treatment plans for patients, referring their patients to EIM-credentialed exercise programs and exercise professionals. Two of the authors of this book (Chris Volgraf and Keith Burns) are EIM credentialed professionals and have worked within this program to help individuals in their communities.

EIM is committed to the belief that physical activity is integral in the prevention and treatments of diseases and should be regularly assessed and "treated" as part of all healthcare. Later in this book, we will break down the process of the ACSM's ground breaking initiative and its effects on preventing disease, managing and rehabilitating diseased populations, and combatting cardiovascular disease.

This book's Strong Heart Fitness Program takes a holistic approach to managing your heart health. We'll be looking at the heart as more than a constantly beating muscle, and will instead be considering it as the emotional life center of the body. Emotions, stress, and physical matter all flow through the heart, and have an effect on its health and recovery. Only by appreciating the heart as part of a larger system, one which benefits from comprehensive approaches to health, can we truly start to see lasting results.

CHAPTER 1

Heart Disease:
What to Know About
Your Condition

According to The American Heart Association, the catch-all term "heart disease" actually describes a number of problems, many of which are related to a process called atherosclerosis. Atherosclerosis is a condition that develops when a substance called plaque builds up in the walls of the arteries. As plaque build-up worsens, the arteries narrow, making it harder for blood to efficiently flow through. If blood clots form, they can completely block the flow of blood, leading to an eventual heart attack or stroke. A heart attack occurs when the blood flow of a coronary artery that supplies a particular area of the heart is blocked by a blood clot. When the clot cuts off blood flow completely in a coronary artery, the area of the heart that receives its blood supply can become necrotic (die).

Although heart attacks can be fatal, many people survive their first heart attack and go on to lead completely normal lives with the help of medications, increased activity levels and modified diets. As with many conditions and injuries, a reoccurrence is highly likely if the patient does not comply with healthy lifestyle changes.

A stroke is sometimes referred to as a "brain attack," as it is similar to a heart attack, but occurs in the brain. Blood clots can form in the brain's blood vessels, in blood vessels leading to the brain, or even in blood vessels throughout the body, breaking away and travelling to the brain. The brain cells impacted by the clot could become injured/impaired or die. Approximately 80 percent of strokes are ischemic strokes, making it the most common form of the event. (A less common form of stroke is a hemopharragic stroke, which occurs when a blood vessel within the brain bursts, often from uncontrollable hypertension or aneurysm.)

If only injured, the brain cells may be rehabilitated to help improve bodily function (speech, movement and memory) and in some cases other brain cells will help perform the "tasks" of the injured cells. Unfortunately, due to the extreme lack of oxygenated blood, some effects of stroke are permanent if too many brain cells die after a stroke.

OTHER TYPES OF CARDIOVASCULAR DISEASE

Heart failure: This type of cardiac disease refers to the heart's inability to keep up with the workload demands of the body. The heart itself does not completely fail, but rather declines in functional capacity. Although there is no cure for this condition, heart failure medications along with positive lifestyle modifications can help the patient lead a normal life.

Arrhythmia: Arrhythmia is the abnormally slow, fast or irregular heart rate rhythm of the heart. Bradycardia refers to a heart rate that is less than 60 beats per minute; tachycardia is a heart rate greater than 100 beats per minute; and an irregular heart rhythm is when the heart beats out of sync, not following a normal pattern. An arrhythmia can affect the heart's function and may not allow the heart to keep up with the body's workload demands. Medications, lifestyle changes, pacemakers, cardioversion and surgery can cure or control the patient's arrhythmia.

Heart valve problems: When heart valves don't open enough to allow the blood to flow through as it should, it's called stenosis. When the heart valves don't close properly and allow blood to leak through, it's called regurgitation. When the valve leaflets bulge or prolapse back into the upper chamber, it's a condition called mitral valve prolapse. When this happens, they may not close properly. This allows blood to flow backward through them.

As you can see, in most cases of heart disease, the disease is both treatable and rehabilitative. When the proper steps are taken, patients can lead not only a normal life, but a healthier and more active life than before their cardiac disease. The thing to remember is…movement *is* medicine!

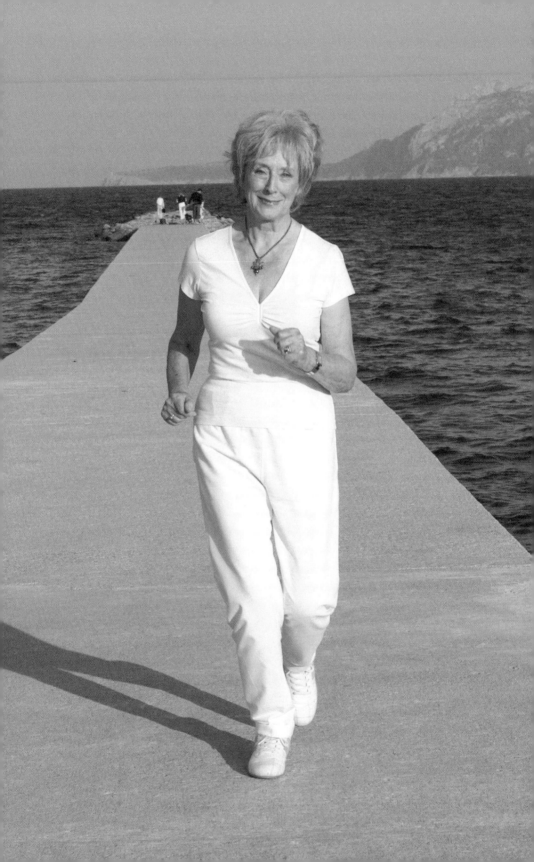

CHAPTER 2

Cardiac Recovery Overview

BASIC HISTORY OF CARDIAC RECOVERY PROGRESS

The phrase "cardiac recovery" likely conjures images of hospital settings—patients walking on treadmills, pedaling on recumbent bikes or using an upper body ergometer. All of this is done for good reason, and is beneficial to the patient's recovery, but here's the catch: what happens to those patients after being discharged from their hospital-based care? That, my friends, is the question of the day, one being hotly debated by everyone from exercise professional to hospital directors.

A major initiative currently taking place in the healthcare industry is looking to prevent wherever possible re-admission of patients back into hospital settings. It makes sense; you wouldn't want to bring your car back into the shop for the same problem you just paid a mechanic to fix. This initiative, known as value-based bundling, began in 2012 with the identification by Medicare of Centers for Excellence (COEs).

COEs are established for health conditions such as joint replacements and congestive heart failure, and are evaluated on their outcome-based care. In other words, they are judged not just on their ability to fix these problems, but their ability to see to it that the problem *stays* fixed.

One of the primary issues in acute care is that, once a patient is discharged, they can either follow the hospital's recommendations for future care (such as continued physical therapy or working with a post-rehabilitation trainer) or they can do nothing at all, depending on their personal level of commitment.

That's where *Exercises for Cardiac Recovery* comes in. Our goal is to help transition patients back to full function after leaving the care of a hospital or other acute care center. Or, in the case of those readers who haven't experience a specific cardiac event, we aim to provide a practical resource to help you get as heart fit as possible.

CARDIAC RECOVERY FIT TIP: WORK-REST RECOVERY

A key design element of any good cardiac fitness program is work-rest ratios. Comprising of frequency, intensity, time, and type, these variables are used by training professionals to progress clients as they get stronger.

- Frequency: times per week
- Intensity: exertion level
- Time: length of activity
- Type: method of exercise

BENEFITS OF A CARDIAC RECOVERY PROGRAM

Let's get down to business. You are reading this book because you want to know how to get your heart and body as strong as possible, and know that the benefits you can expect to see from regular participation in a cardiac recovery program will keep you motivated and focused.

During a cardiac event, heart tissue is damaged. Scar tissue, lingering damage to the neurology (i.e. circuitry) of the heart, or weakening of valves (resulting in regurgitation) are all examples of potential after-effects of a cardiac episode. To strength the heart and address these deficiencies, the prudent approach (i.e. the approach utilized by the majority of private and public health care services) is to recommend patients follow the best practice exercise protocols per nationally recognized certifying bodies such as the American College of Sports Medicine or the National Strength and Conditioning Association.

But for most of us, because 80 percent of care occurs outside medical supervision, our hearts continue to weaken over time. So, it would be wise for anyone looking to participate in a heart healthy program to actively pursue resources that not only strengthen the heart but also teach the body to move more efficiently.

LONGEVITY: STRENGTHENING THE HEART FOR BETTER NUTRIENT DELIVERY

It's undeniable that, due to advances in the field of medicine, pharmaceuticals, and a better understanding of the importance of nutrition and exercise, people are generally living longer. But does living longer mean we are living better?

A strong argument can be made that, due to poor behavioral and lifestyle choices (primarily associated with changes in the workforce dynamic), the aforementioned advancements fail to offset the ill effects of an increasingly sedentary population. Between working, sleeping and family/life commitments, the average person is left with very little time for physical activity. This is why good heart health habits are so vital and are often stressed by healthcare providers as the key to achieving sustained well-being and high quality of life. Every little bit *does* count; what you eat for breakfast, that walk you take at lunch, the quality of your sleep, and a healthy home and work life all contribute, for good or ill, to your health. When being healthy is not a priority, bad daily habits set in, which can lead to weeks, months or even years of poor lifestyle choices.

THE BIG PICTURE: HEALTH-RELATED PHYSICAL FITNESS

The Strong Heart Fitness Program in this book will certainly improve your cardiac function, and while that is the primary *focus* of this book, it would not do to overlook the other components of fitness that we seek to improve as part of a complete prevention and recovery plan.

These components (based on ACSM's Guidelines for Exercise Testing and Prescription) include:

- Cardiovascular endurance: the ability to sustain aerobic physical activity
- Body composition: percentage of the body that is muscle, fat, bone
- Muscle strength: the ability to exert force
- Muscle endurance: the ability to perform without fatigue
- Flexibility: the body's range of motion

CREATING A SAFE EXERCISE PRESCRIPTION

In order to help patients achieve progress and improvement in the fitness components listed above, the fitness professional's number one job is to establish a safe and effective program. The fitness professional must take the patients' health history, most recent medical exam outcomes and current diagnosis into consideration when setting up the safest exercise program possible.

The following are some things that should be taken into account when designing a safe and effective exercise program.

Clinical Status

This is prerequisite to get the process started for low to high risk patients. Has the patient successfully completed supervised Phase III Cardiac Rehab? Have they received a physician's clearance to start and participate in an exercise program (one prescribed by a degreed and certified health professional)?

Risk Stratification

The ACSM place patients in one of three levels of risk stratification, based on their age and preexisting cardiovascular risk factors. These risk factors include:

CORONARY ARTERY DISEASE: RISK FACTOR THRESHOLDS	
Family History	Myocardial infarction, coronary revascularization, or sudden death before 55 years of age in father or other male of first degree relationship (either brother or son), or before 65 years of age in mother or other female first degree relative (either sister or daughter)
Cigarette Smoking	Current cigarette smoker or one who quit within the previous 6 months
Hypertension	Systolic blood pressure of 140 mmHg and higher, or diastolic of 90 mmHg and higher, confirmed by measurements on at least two separate occasions; or, currently on antihypertensive medication
Hypercholesterolemia	Total serum cholesterol greater than 200 mg/dL or high-density lipoprotein cholesterol less than 35 mg/dL; or, on lipid-lowering medication. If low-density lipoprotein cholesterol is available, use greater than 130 mg/dL rather than total cholesterol greater than 200 mg/dL.
Impaired Fasting Glucose	Fasting blood glucose greater than or equal to 110/ mg/dL, confirmed by measurements on at least two separate occasions
Obesity	Body Mass Index greater than or equal to 30 kg/m^2, or waist girth greater than 100 cm
Sedentary Lifestyle	Persons not participating in a regular exercise program or meeting the minimal physical activity recommendations from the U.S. Surgeon General's report
High Serum HDL Cholesterol	Greater than 60 mg/dL

ACSM's Guidelines for Exercise Testing and Prescription, 8th Edition, 2010

After assessing an individual based on these criteria, the ACSM will then place them in one of three categories:

Low Risk. Young individuals who are asymptomatic and meet no more than one risk factor threshold.

Moderate Risk. Older individuals (men older than 45 years of and women older than 55 years of age) who meet the threshold for two or more risk factors.

High Risk. Individuals with one or more signs/symptoms listed in the Coronary Artery Disease Risk Factor table, or who are known to have cardiovascular, pulmonary or metabolic disease.

CARDIAC RECOVERY FIT TIP:
CARDIAC HEALTH IS MORE THAN A TREADMILL TEST
Cardiac health in measured in a number of ways. Many readers may have experienced a stress test in their cardiologist's office. This is a physical test based around specific parameters including heart rate response, blood pressure, and RPE. However, "field tests"—that is, tests you administer yourself during normal conditions—are generally more practical if you want to establish your own heart health baseline. To perform, go to your local high school track and measure out a distance of 1 mile. Record the time it takes you to complete the 1-mile distance. Make note of your heart rate at the start, end and 3 minutes after completion.

Results of Exercise Stress Test

Cardiovascular patients of moderate to high risk undergo a sub-maximal or maximal treadmill stress test to determine their exercise capacity. This test will also determine a safe exercise intensity (measured in heart rate, blood pressure or rate of perceived exertion) for the patient, one free of ischemic ECG changes and physical symptoms.

Medications

The presence of medications such as beta blockers (used to treat hypertension) can attenuate the heart rate at rest and during exercise. This will change the exercise prescription in regards to heart rate and blood pressure.

Comorbidities

While cardiovascular disease is our primary focus, there are situations when a patient presents with one or more additional diseases, aside from cardiovascular disease. The disease or disorder does not necessarily need to be associated or related to CV (such as diabetes mellitus); it can also be mental or behavioral in origin.

Orthopedic Concerns

Preexisting injuries and physical conditions or degeneration of the musculoskeletal system, connective tissues and joints may make it necessary to modify a patient's program design. For example, a patient with progressive osteoarthritis may not be able to tolerate the impact of treadmill walking; therefore, their cardiovascular exercise prescription may need to be performed on a stationary bike or similar modality.

History of Physical Activity

Sedentary patients and active patients will have different needs in regards to professional supervision. Sedentary individuals will need to be treated with greater supervision due to their unfamiliarity with different bodily movement patterns (squats, hinges, presses, etc.) and exercise equipment. Not only are sedentary individuals at greater risk of physical injury (as the ACSM risk stratification states), their risk only increases if they are obese.

CARDIOVASCULAR EXERCISE RECOMMENDATIONS FOR CARDIAC RECOVERY

The ACSM also provides recommendations on the Frequency, Intensity, Time and Type of exercise (FITT Principle) to help prevent, manage and rehabilitate cardiovascular disease. These recommendations are based on years of medical research and observed outcomes.

Frequency

The American College of Sports Medicine recommends exercising 4–7 days per week to facilitate cardiovascular fitness and improved body composition.

Goals may include:

- Increasing number of days per week spent physically active and/or engaging in regular exercise
- Engaging in supervised PLUS home exercise routines

Intensity

The ACSM promotes the following methods for prescribing and monitoring exercise intensity:

- Heart Rate Reserve (HRR)
- Workload (METs)
- Rating of Perceived Exertion (RPE)
- Heart Rate Method (HR)

Of these, this book will be using the Heart Rate Reserve Method, in accordance with the newest American College of Sports Medicine guidelines (explained below). Regardless of the method used, intensity needs to be above minimal levels, while remaining below the metabolic load that evokes abnormal clinical signs/symptoms. In other words, avoiding myocardial ischemia or arrhythmias (10–15 beats per minute below standard) and any symptoms of angina.

Rating of Perceived Exertion. While performing a sustained level of physical activity, the individual is asked to assign a numerical value to their level of general fatigue and stress, with 1 being a low score (extremely easy, virtually no exertion perceived) and 20 being nearly impossible (requiring everything they have to perform the movement).

THR Methods. The Training Heart Rate (THR) method generally relies on one of two statistics:

- Percent of Heart Rate Reserve (HRR)
- Percent of heart rate max (HR max)

Heart rate reserve (HRR) is the difference between resting heart rate (HRrest) and maximum heart rate (HRmax).

$$HRR = HRmax - HRrest.$$

Percent of heart rate max (HRmax) is determined by taking the patient's max heart rate (generally found by subtracting the patient's age from 220) and taking 75–85 percent of that figure to find the optimal intensity for exercise training. For those less fit, a lower THR may be more appropriate (around 50–70 percent).

Time

In regards to use of time when determining an exercise program, the ACSM generally recommends the following guidelines:

- A warm up/cooldown period (approximately 5–10 minutes) at less than 40 percent HRR or an RPE between 9–11
- 20–60 minutes of continuous or intermittent aerobic activity, with duration varying inversely to intensity

CARDIAC RECOVERY FIT TIP: ACTIVE RECOVERY

Active recovery refers to following a vigorous activity with a low intensity activity; for example, fast power walking followed by a half speed walk. Activity recovery assists with lowering heart rate and breathing rate slowly, prevents dizziness occurring from abrupt stopping, and decreases acidic build-up in muscles. Never stop abruptly after a strenuous exertion—always keep moving.

Type of Exercise

Cardiovascular exercise includes activities such as walking, incline walking, cycling, elliptical training, rowing, jogging, running, and swimming.

In terms of resistance training, cardiac patients are recommended to engage in resistance training 2–3 days a week, performing 10–15 reps (working to mild muscle fatigue) of 8–10 exercises that address the major muscle groups.

Flexibility exercises should also be incorporated into the overall fitness program at levels sufficient to develop and maintain target range of motion. These exercises should stretch the major muscle groups and be performed a minimum of 2–3 days a week. This can include appropriate static stretches (to the point of mild discomfort). Each static stretch should be held for 10–30 seconds and repeated up to 3–4 times.

BENEFITS OF WALKING

There are few activities that as healthy and easy to implement into your daily life as a walking routine. The health benefits of walking include (but are certainly not limited to):

Manages your weight. Combined with healthy eating, physical activity is key to long-lasting weight control. Keeping your weight within healthy limits can lower your risks of type 2 diabetes, heart disease, stroke, cancer, sleep apnea, and osteoarthritis.

Controls your blood pressure. Physical activity strengthens the heart, so it can pump more blood with less effort and with less pressure on the arteries. Staying fit is just as effective as some medications in keeping blood pressure levels low.

Decreases your risk of heart attack. Exercise, such as brisk walking for three hours a week, or just half an hour a day, is associated with a 30–40 percent lower risk of heart disease in women.

Boosts "good" cholesterol (high-density lipoproteins or HDL). Physical activity helps reduce low-density lipoproteins (LDL or "bad" cholesterol) in the blood, which can cause plaque buildup along the artery walls, a major cause of heart attacks.

Lowers your risk of stroke. Regular, moderate exercise equivalent to brisk walking for an hour a day, five days a week, can cut the risk of stroke in half, according to a Harvard study of more than 11,000 men.

Reduces your risk of breast cancer and Type 2 diabetes. The Nurses' Health Study also links regular activity to risk reductions for both diseases. In another study, people at high risk of diabetes cut their risk in half by combining consistent exercise, like walking, with lower fat intake and a 5–7 percent weight loss.

Reduces need for gallstone surgery. Regular walking or other physical activity lowers the risk of needing gallstone surgery by 20–31 percent, found a Harvard study of more than 60,000 women ages 40–65.

Protects against hip fracture. Consistent activity diminishes the risk of hip fracture, concludes a study of more than 30,000 men and women ages 20–93.

Other studies have suggested a daily brisk walk can also help prevent depression, colon cancer, osteoporosis, and impotence. In addition, walks may lengthen lifespan, lower stress levels, relieve arthritis and back pain, strengthen muscles, bones and joints, improve sleep, and elevate mood and sense of well-being.

How can you go wrong with walking once a day? Try it for two weeks and keep a journal about where you walk and how you feel before/after the walk. Make note of your fitness level before the two weeks, and afterwards.

Remember to keep a steady routine by walking for at least 30 minutes a day, five or more days a week to get the most out of your program. Make the walks fun too—bring a friend, walk your dog, or listen to music. And as always, be sure to consult your doctor first before starting any exercise program!

—Contributed by Angela Pappano, MS, NCC and UC Berkeley, Women's Health letter)

HABITS: THE GOOD, BAD AND UGLY

Exercises for Cardiac Recovery stresses the need for good daily habits. To that end, we have dedicated an entire section to incorporating good heart health habits into your daily routine. Think of these as choices to be made on auto-pilot; once you can perform these habits without hesitation, you'll have come a long way towards improving your health.

Practicing good health habits lets you...

- Decrease the chance of relapse
- Stay out of the hospital
- Increase functional status (especially for the aging/elderly population)

Elements of Cardiac Wellness

Social Wellness. It may seem surprising, but maintaining an adequately stimulating and fulfilling social life serves to lay the foundation for a whole-body approach to heart health. By making sure that you stay active and engaged in your daily life, you not only avoid some of the unpleasant mental and emotional obstacles (like depression or persistent anxiety) which can interfere with your recovery, you enable yourself to stay motivated to improve. A good way to get yourself out there in a positive way is to volunteer in your community, which helps keep you current and involved in your environment.

Mental Wellness. The hope is that by working to improve your social wellness, your mental and emotional wellness will follow suit. Try to find activities that provide you with stress-free enjoyment, as well as hobbies that allow you a defense mechanism for stress relief. Dealing with cardiac illness and working towards full recovery can be challenging, even discouraging at times. But by making sure to focus on triggering that rush of endorphins that comes with having a good time, you keep yourself in the right state of mind and keep yourself moving forward.

Physical Wellness. Staying active and stress-free won't do much if you're neglecting your physical wellness. That said, just by picking up this book you've demonstrated that you're willing to commit to preserving and improving your physical well-being. This includes following all your doctor's recommendations, staying committed to your recovery program, working through your exercise progressions, and fueling your body with the proper nutrition and supplements.

When all three of these elements of your health are balanced, you achieve the sort of whole-body well-being that everyone should aspire to.

MIND-BODY CONNECTION

Popularizing the "mind-body" approach to medicine, Dr. Herbert Benson saw the link between chronic diseases—including heart disease, hypertension, and intestinal discomfort—to stress and the inflammatory response of the body.

Dr. Benson also commented on the importance of social and communal elements in our lives and their role as precursors to developing risk factors. Research into the mind-body approach has shown that positive reinforcement or altering thought processes (cognitive-behavioral therapy), relaxation therapy (para-sympathetic nervous responses), and self-care (engaging one's health with evidence-based self-therapy) have protective effects on your health.

So, why are we discussing this in a book on cardiac recovery? As Dr. Benson demonstrated in his stress response studies, the path to chronic disease can develop from environmental, vocational, and ultimately controllable factors. Many of these are the same risk factors that cause increased stress and cardiac difficulties.

Using the chart on page xx, develop your own Healthy Mind Map to help you identify the various factors impacting your cardiac health, ultimately helping you control these factors.

Support from Family Members: Oftentimes, the ones closest to you either can hinder or accelerate your path towards health. Having those closest to you in support of your new healthy lifestyle is crucial. Ask yourself whether you have been more or less likely to be active because of your spouse's or relative's attitudes towards exercise.

Stress: Stress can present itself in good ways (such as a job promotion) or bad ways (for instance, experiencing financial difficulties). Controlling stress through meditation, time management techniques, or healthy eating are a few strategies that can prevent stress from complicating your rehabilitation.

Journaling: Spend a few minutes each day writing down which activities you did and how you felt before and after that activity. This can help you identify which activities are placing stress on your body.

Lifestyle: Nutrition, smoking, waist circumference, and inactivity are several examples of controllable risk factors that can make you more susceptible to cardiac arrest.

Support from Doctors and Therapists: Keep an open dialogue—if your therapist knows the lifestyle factors affecting your cardiac health, they will be better able to guide you towards more beneficial health habits.

Exercise Therapy: The exercises in this book will help you build a strong foundation for managing your cardiac recovery process, but further treatment with a physical therapist may be beneficial in some cases and necessary in others.

TRANSITIONING BACK TO FUNCTIONAL STATUS

The experience of transitioning out of a hospital-based care setting back into the community (and, ultimately, into your home) has changed quite a bit in the last five years. There are three reasons that come to mind that explain this:

Value-based medicine initiatives. Providers and health systems are working more closely than ever with insurance carriers to tie reimbursements back to the actual outcomes of patients. By providing more value to the patient in the form of improved health and management, providers thus receive a share of the savings incurred from keeping the patient healthier. An example would be a patient with congestive heart complications being managed on an outpatient basis, rather than being re-admitted for the same condition. Well-managed health systems will often try to ensure physicians are following best-practices by acquiring the practice, employing the doctor, and aligning them to expected patient outcomes. These efforts get everyone on the same team—*your* team.

Population health. This concept reflects a community-focused approach. In this model, health systems are essentially assigned large groups of people to manage and given a per-member fee to keep these people healthy. For example, Medicare may assign certain healthcare systems 100,000 Medicare patients drawn from a large area in your state. That system is paid the fee plus incentives if high risk patients are managed aggressively. In your doctor's office, you'll likely receive on-going calls from a nurse asking about your medications, exercise regimen, symptoms, and related healthy living parameters.

Centers of Excellence. A Center of Excellence (COE) is established around a certain condition, which could be anything from orthopedics to cardiology. The COE then aligns associated hospitals, doctors and supporting care providers with expected outcomes, compensation systems and managed care integration for long-term best practice for the specific condition. This health system understands that if they manage a patient effectively with evidence-based medicine, they minimize cost, ease the transition to outpatient care, and prevent readmission longer than a defined period. Their shared savings will then be higher than if the patient was re-admitted for, say, an infection tied to the procedure.

As for what has motivated these recent changes, Medicare tends to drive a lot of the updates that take place in the commercial insurance markets. Because of the way health insurance markets were set up, physicians were previously being compensated on a fee-for-service model of compensation. Essentially, the more services they provided, the more they were paid, rather than the resulting health of the patient guiding the compensation.

Seems backwards, right?

CREATING A SOCIAL SUPPORT SYSTEM

Establishing a network of close relationships for a patient in cardiac recovery is an excellent strategy that will support their physical and mental rehabilitation.

Getting out of the house and meeting people should be the first step. We know that isolation from others can lead to depression, which in turn results in a lapse in following one's recovery protocol. In addition, endorphins (a.k.a. the body's natural pain medication) are released through fulfilling, happy experiences; by engaging friendly and caring individuals, we reinforce the healthy neural connections needed for new lifestyle habits, creating positive reinforcement for healthy behavior.

Establishing a Network of Professional Caregivers

In addition to friends and family, professionals that have extensive experience and knowledge-based intellect in the field of cardiac recovery are vital. This is hardly an all-inclusive list, so please refer to your primary care provider for additional information.

Primary Care Physician

Primary care practitioners are coming back into vogue. The "medical home" model, in which the emphasis lies on a personal physician in a long-term medical relationship with the patient, and who is therefore capable of acute, chronic and continuous comprehensive care, is re-empowering the original providers of medical care. The trend over the last couple of decades has drifted away from the primary care doctor towards specialists that order expensive tests and scans. Having one point of contact is key to coordinating patient care.

Psychologist or Psychiatrist

The mental aspects of cardiac recovery, and of any lengthy recovery process, are more numerous and impactful than many might suspect. Knowing and appreciating the need for mental support during cardiac recovery will benefit you in the long run, and so having access to a mental healthcare professional on your support team is vital.

Social Worker

An experienced social worker can coordinate family and friends, along with the necessary medical care. Social workers become an integral part of the familial structure when there has been an injury or acute medical incident (stroke, fall, etc.) that has led to the patient becoming disabled.

Physical and/or Occupational Therapist

Clinical rehabilitation (pain free, range of motion) and restoring function are the initial objectives or a physical or occupational therapist. Their next goal is to establish an exercise program that can be taken with the patient following treatment.

For caregivers, help your patient or loved one get their day back on track with these nine tips to help smooth out the ups and downs in their daily schedule:

Stretch for 5 minutes before getting out of bed in the morning to prepare your muscles for movement.

Drink one large glass of water in the morning to stabilize your morning eating habits. Our bodies are approximately 60% water. By replenishing our body first thing in the morning, the regulatory systems of our body, namely heart rate and blood pressure, will stay increasingly balanced.

Eat 300-400 calories for breakfast. Starting the day off right with a healthy breakfast keeps our energy levels balanced throughout the day.

Healthy lunch foods can easily be made to order at local restaurants. Pick steamed and broiled foods over fried. Gastrointestinal (GI) irritability can be exacerbated by fried and processed foods.

Mid-afternoon is a perfect time to have **a moderate carbohydrate/moderate protein-based snack or drink.** An example would be a smoothie of dark berries with whey protein blended with water. Martha Raidl, a nutrition specialist at the University of Idaho Extension Program suggests beverages like plain or flavored water, or iced or hot tea as long as it's unsweetened. If this doesn't satisfy you, try a 100-calorie snack.

Early dinners around 5:00 or 6:00 can be on the heavier side, whereas dinners at 7:00 or later should be on the lighter side. If you know your dinner will be later, add another serving of milk instead of water to your smoothie, increasing the total caloric intake for your mid-afternoon snack.

Take a walk after dinner, but wait 20-30 minutes after eating. Stimulating blood flow through aerobically-based movements that are low impact (not running) aids in the digestive process. Giving 30 minutes allows the food to settle.

Write a short to-do list before going to bed. Keep your list to 3 priority items if you do not work and 1-2 priority items if you have a full-time occupation.

Practice deep breathing as a form of relaxation before bed. Deep breathing is an excellent way to slow the heart rate. Focus on breathing in through the nose and out through the mouth.

Fitness Professional (Personal Trainer)

As a physical trainer, this category is dear to my heart! The personal trainer is the frontline of prevention. Listening, interpersonal communication skills, and knowledge-based skills are absolutes for quality personal trainers. Solid trainers have an excellent repertoire with medical providers and colleagues in the fitness community.

Personal trainers are also better equipped to provide care that respects the feelings of people in cardiac recovery, helping them to make the most of their existing capacity to work towards achievable, practical health goals.

CHAPTER 3

Assessment
and Screening

efore getting into a general overview of the most common heart-related issues, it's vital that the reader remember the scope of this book. This book is focused on those people who have been advised by their doctor to continue with an exercise program post-cardiac rehab or after being diagnosed with heart disease. Moving forward, we will assume that you are stable and have been cleared for exercises.

The Strong Heart Fitness Program is designed to be progressively challenging, incorporating more muscle groups, more movement with greater workloads, and less rest, as time goes on. The team of professional trainers writing this resource has designed these programs as if you were their own clients. With this in mind, we've taken great pains to prepare a comprehensive program, one designed to take the whole body into consideration, with the heart and its health at the center of everything.

CARDIAC RECOVERY RISK FACTORS

When targeting cardiac health and cardiac recovery through exercise, it is important to understand the risk factors involved. Thankfully, many of these risk factors can be controlled (or else mitigated) through healthy daily habits.

Examples of controllable risk factors include:

- Your Body Mass Index (BMI)
- Your waist-to-hip circumference
- Your percentage body fat
- Your overall physical activity levels
- Diet and nutrition
- Nutritional supplements

Examples of chronic or uncontrollable conditions to keep in mind include:

- Risk of congestive heart failure
- Risk of heart attack
- Electrophysiology (the way your body's wired)
- Acute conditions which inhibit physical activity
- Pre-existing congenital conditions

PRE-EXISTING CONGENITAL CONDITIONS

Before beginning any exercise program, it's important to establish a baseline. This baseline provides you with a foundation to interpret on-going feedback on your progress. Thankfully, the world of human movement science includes a seemingly endless variety of screenings, tests and evaluations that can provide useful data, tailored to the specific audience.

In the case of heart disease, the reader will henceforth be understood to have gone through an extensive medical exam with a medical doctor or cardiologist, including recent blood lab results and a physical work up (including a sub max or maximal stress test). The results of these exams are what determine whether a patient is cleared for physical activity—which, as stated at the beginning of this book, will be assumed going forward.

Activities of Daily Living (ADLs)

In this assessment, we make some basic assumptions, owing to the fact that our readers are generally healthy and able to perform basic activities of daily living. With that said, for those of our readers who may have physical limitations, it is important to establish baselines.

Perform these movements as a baseline comparison for activities performed throughout your daily routine.

Basic ADLs: Basic ADLs are those tasks we perform on a daily basis. How many of the following can you complete without difficulty?

- Bathing
- Dressing
- Self-feeding
- Personal hygiene and grooming
- Toilet hygiene

Instrumental ADLs: Instrumental ADLs are slightly more complex uses of the body's functional mobility, and typically involve multiple basic ADLs being used simultaneously. Postural conditions can impact one's ability to perform these activities of daily living. For example, the inability to raise one's arm above their head due to rounded shoulders or kyphosis prohibits one from being able to place dishes in a cabinet. Or, a limited ability to bend over (with proper squat mechanics) without low back pain makes it much more difficult to pick something up off the floor.

ACTIVATING THE RELAXATION RESPONSE

Take a deep breath into your belly, and count to five. Pause for one second, then breathe out slowly to another count of five. Remember to keep your belly soft. Repeat this routine five times, and perform this exercise daily to benefit from the cumulative effect of daily practice.

This exercise is one of many that can be performed to activate your vagus nerve, which extends from your brain through your neck down through your diaphragm. When you breathe deeply, it stimulates the parasympathetic nervous system to create that 'relaxation response' we all yearn to achieve. (Now you know why trainers, Pilates and yoga instructors, and therapists all want you to breathe during exercise!)

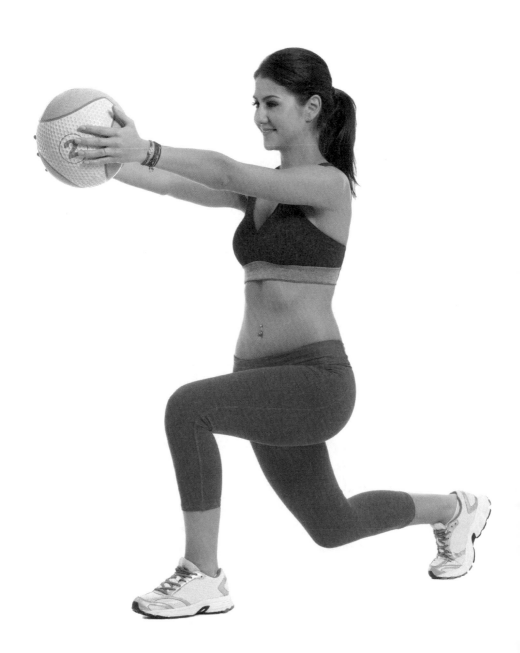

CHAPTER 4

The Exercises

I n selecting the perfect exercises to aid in both general and targeted cardiac recovery, we've chosen to prioritize a holistic approach, where possible. The exercises contained in this book take into account the fact that the heart is part of a much larger system—the human body—that is constantly in need of oxygen and nutrients. Think about it: when you walk up the stairs while de-conditioned, what happens? After an initially delayed response, your heart rate begins to rise, your breathing rate increases and, if it's a long staircase, you may even experience acute muscle fatigue. If you stop abruptly at the top, you're likely due for a bit of acute dizziness from blood pooling in your local extremities.

While you'll likely return to a resting state after 1–2 minutes, this example illustrates why the heart is just a piece—albeit the most important piece—a larger puzzle, one comprised of muscles, joints, fascia and countless other structures. When performing the exercises in our Strong Heart Fitness Program, you may not feel like you are strictly training the heart. But this is exactly what we want. A strong heart is the center of a strong body. With that in mind, we will be working your legs, hips, core, and shoulder girdle. Your posture will improve as you begin to stand more upright, allowing the lungs to expand and contract without restriction. Your calf muscles will get stronger, allowing for better balance and enhanced circulation back to the heart, thereby decreasing recovery time between exercises.

The exercises were purposely selected with an eye towards balancing all three planes of movement: frontal (side to side), sagittal (front to back), and transverse (rotational). By working these planes individually or in combination, we allow for a never ending selection of program possibilities, as well as countless exercises to choose from.

Think of Strong Heart Fitness Program as a "NON-Cardiac Recovery" resource. We're "buffing" your heart to better improve its function, and the function of all its related systems.

Many of the exercises in this program can be modified or further improved by the use of standard gym equipment. For a full list of recommended gym equipment for each exercise, please see the table at the end of this book.

Band Pull Apart

FEEL IT HERE: upper back, shoulders, arms

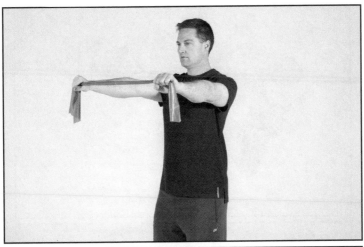

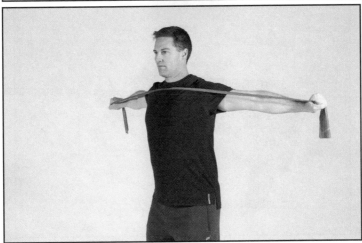

Place a shortened band in hands with arms extended out in front of the body. Slowly retract the shoulder blades, pulling the band apart until the arms reach the sides of the body in a full range of motion. Return slowly to starting position. Perform 10–15 reps.

Dumbbell Chest Press

FEEL IT HERE: chest, shoulders, arms

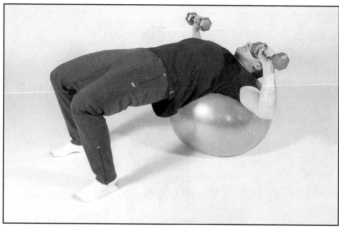

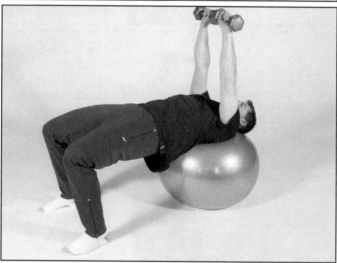

This exercise can be completed on a bench or using a physioball for an increasingly difficult exercise. Position feet slightly wider than the hips and keep feet firm on the floor. Bring the dumbbells down to a position in front of the shoulders. Push the dumbbells back up in an alternating pattern, following an outside/inside path.

Spiderman

FEEL IT HERE: legs, hips, shoulders, core

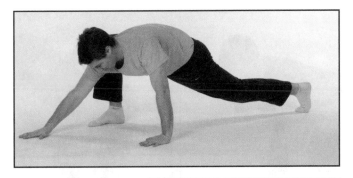

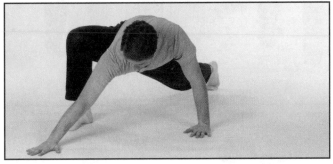

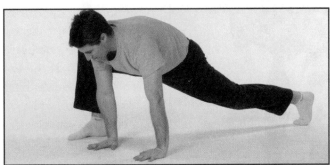

Assume a lunging position. Allow the opposite side hand to come forward with the opposite side foot. Gently rock back and forth before repeating the movement on the other side."

Dumbbell Rows

FEEL IT HERE: upper/middle back, shoulders, arms

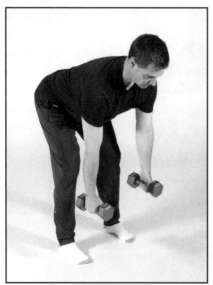

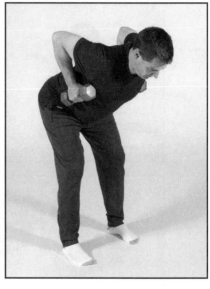

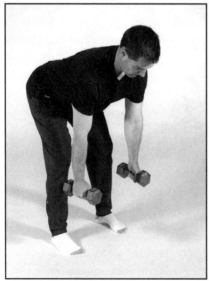

Grab dumbbells at about shoulder width apart. Adopt a deadlift position (lower back neutral, bent over at the waist, knees slightly bent) until the dumbbells are at knee height. Start the exercise by pulling your shoulder blades back, holding in place, while pulling the dumbbells to your sides."

Dumbbell Overhead Press

FEEL IT HERE: shoulders, core, arms

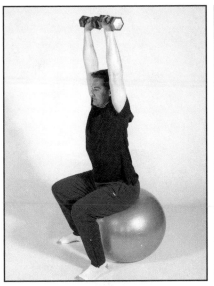

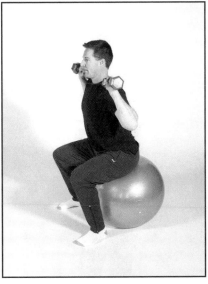

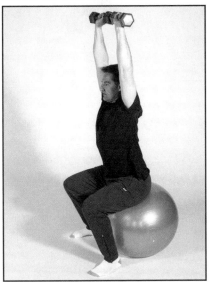

Standing, hold a pair of dumbbells at shoulder height with an overhand grip, about shoulder width apart. Start the movement by pushing the dumbbells vertically over your head until your arms are fully extended. Lower the dumbbells back to the shoulders after your arms have reached full extension.

Dumbbell Squat

FEEL IT HERE: core, hips, legs

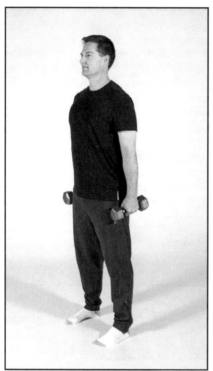 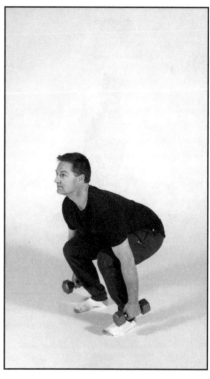

Extend two dumbbells above your head and stabilize. Squat to your lowest depth while maintaining a neutral spine, knees over the outside threes toes, and as a vertical shin as possible. Once you have reached a safe depth, drive your feet into the ground, keep your chest up and push your hips forward.

Bicep Curl to Shoulder Press
FEEL IT HERE: arms, shoulders

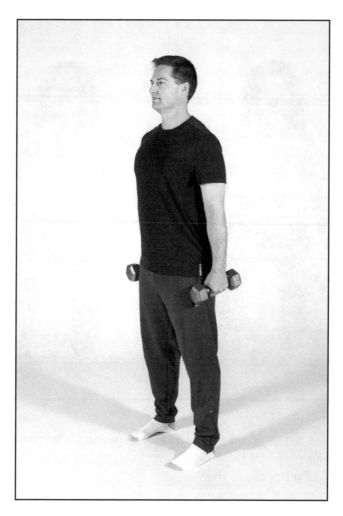

Position the feet under the hips and brace your core. The first part of this movement involves curling the dumbbells to the shoulders. Then, rotate the dumbbells to a neutral shoulder position and follow with a press above the head

35

Bicep Curls

FEEL IT HERE: arms

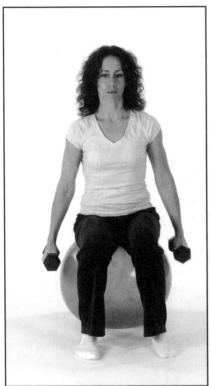 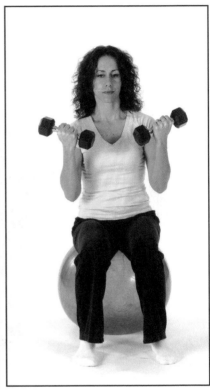

This exercise can be completed on a bench or using a physioball. Position the feet slightly wider than the hips and keep feet firmly on the floor. Curl both dumbbells up to the shoulders simultaneously.

Body Weight Squat

FEEL IT HERE: core, hips, legs

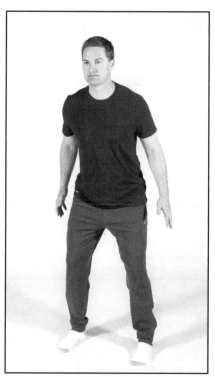 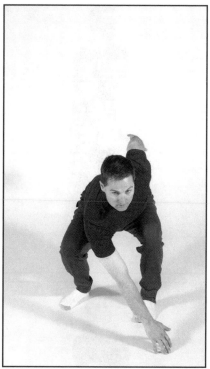

Keeping your arms raised and extended in front of your eyes, stand with your feet about shoulder width apart and toes straight ahead. Initiate the exercise by pushing your hips back with a neutral lower back, allowing your knees to bend naturally. Attempt to maintain a vertical shin as you squat down and pause for 2 seconds. Drive your heels into the ground to push yourself back up.

Dumbbell Deadlifts

FEEL IT HERE: core, hips, legs

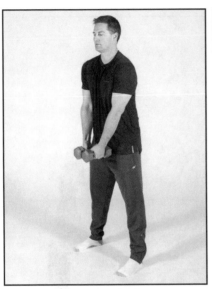
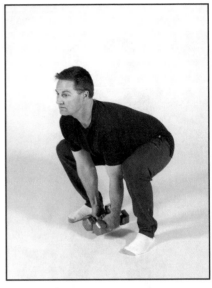
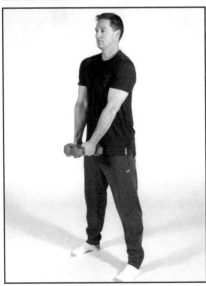

Grab dumbbells with an over-hand grip, about shoulder width apart. Pull your shoulder blades down and back, slightly bending your knees. Initiate the movement by pushing your hips back while keeping your chest up to lower the dumbbells towards the floor. Lower the dumbbells as much as you can (mid-shin is the goal) while feeling a good stretch in the hamstrings and keeping a neutral spine. At the bottom position your chest should be slightly in front of the dumbbells. Finish by tightening your glutes and standing up.

Dumbbell Double Arm Row

FEEL IT HERE: arms, shoulders, back

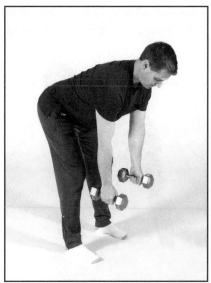
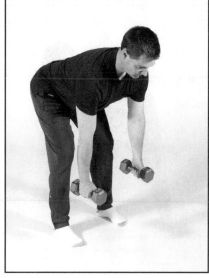

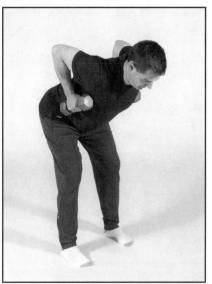

While seated, grab two dumbbells and assume a deadlift position (lower back neutral, bent over at the waist, knees slightly bent). Initiate the exercise by pulling your shoulder blades down and back while pulling the dumbbells up, keeping the elbows close to the body.

Dumbbell Single Arm Row

FEEL IT HERE: arms, shoulders, back

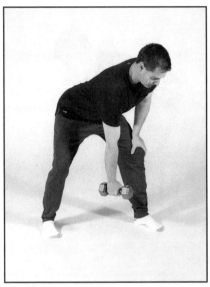 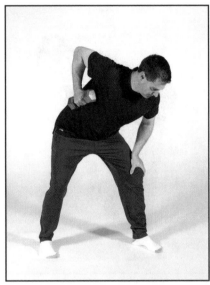

Grab a dumbbell and assume a deadlift position (lower back neutral, bent over at the waist, knees slightly bent). Place the hand without a dumbbell on your hip. Initiate the exercise by pulling your shoulder blades down and back while pulling the dumbbell up, keeping the elbow close to your body. Using only one dumbbell forces the body to use more core stability to maintain proper form.

Saws

FEEL IT HERE: upper back

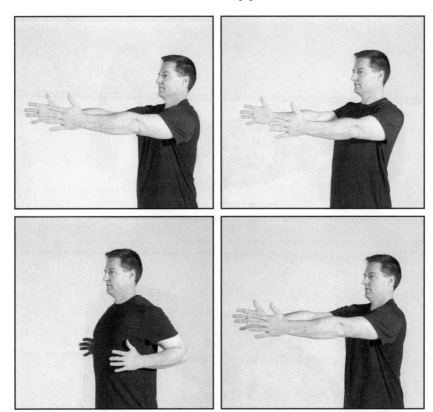

Stand in an upright position with your arms extended in front of your body with palms facing in. Pull the shoulder blades back and bring the arms towards the body, to your full range of motion. Squeeze the upper back muscles, stabilizing the shoulder blades momentarily, before extending arms back to the starting position. Perform 1–2 sets of 10–15 reps. Progressions for saws include performing the motion with palms down, or with thumbs down.

Glute Bridge

FEEL IT HERE: legs, hips, back

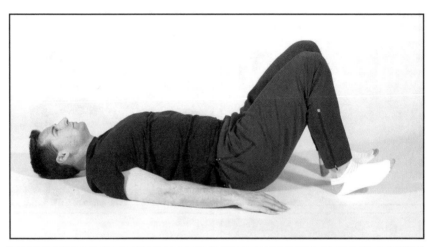

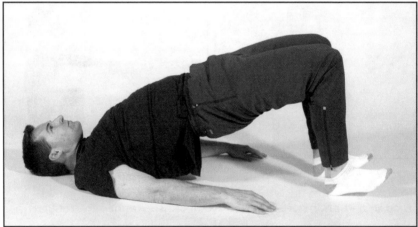

Lying supine with your knees bent and feet flat on the floor, contract your glutes and raise your hips off the floor until your body is in a straight line. Perform 1–3 sets of 10–15 repetitions.

Progress to a Single Leg Hip Bridge, then to performing the bridging action with feet on a physio/stability ball.

Goblet Squat

FEEL IT HERE: legs, hips, back

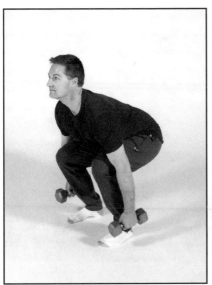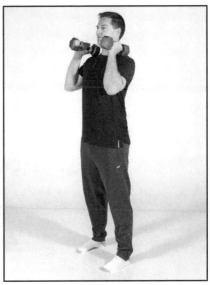

Standing, hold one kettlebell or dumbbell under your chin with your elbows pointing down, feet about shoulder width apart, toes straight ahead. Start by pushing your hips back with a neutral lower back, allowing your knees to bend naturally. Attempt to maintain a vertical shin as you squat down until your quads are parallel to the ground. Pause for 2 seconds, and then drive your heels into the ground to push yourself back up. The weight is used to keep your posture more upright and teach better squat depth.

You can also incorporate a shoulder press into this motion. As you push yourself back up, bring the kettlebell or dumbbell vertically over your head until your arms are fully extended. Lower the weight back down as you return to the starting position.

Incline Dumbbell Chest Press
FEEL IT HERE: chest, shoulders, arms

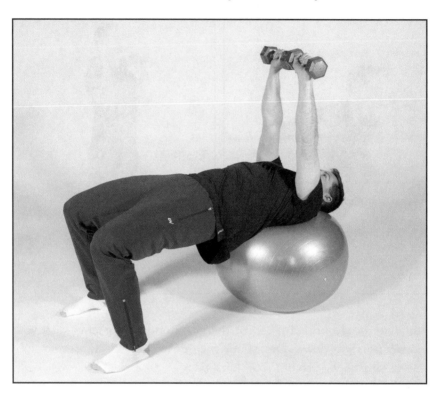

Using the incline position on a bench, position feet slightly wider than the hips and keep feet firmly on the floor. Bring the dumbbells down to a position in front of the shoulders. Push the dumbbells back up following an outside/inside path.

This exercise can also be performed using a bench for greater stability.

Upright Row with Band
FEEL IT HERE: upper back, shoulders

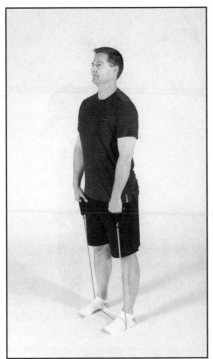 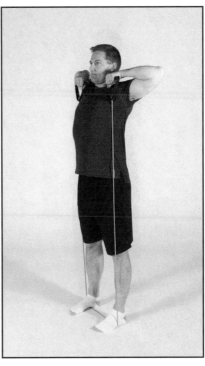

Assume a split stance with band grips in hand and band anchored in front of you. Back up to an appropriate distance to create challenging resistance with arms extended. Retract shoulder blades, pulling your hands towards your nose to full range of motion in the shoulder blades. Return the band back to starting position. Perform 10–15 reps.

Progressions include using a rope or cable attachment with a supine/internal rotation grip.

Draw the Sword

FEEL IT HERE: arms, shoulders, upper back

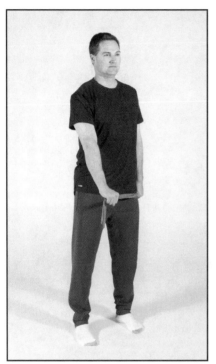 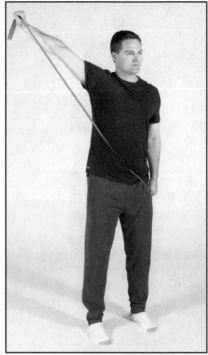

Stand with soft knees and the abdominals drawn in. Start with your arm across your body next to the opposite hip/pocket. Keeping the elbow fixed, pull the arm up and across the body slowly, externally rotating the arm so that the thumb is pointing behind you at the top of the movement with the arm above the head. Return to starting position and repeat 10–15 times.

Progressions for Draw the Sword include using no weight, a light dumbbell or a light resistance band.

Lateral Raise

FEEL IT HERE: shoulders, upper back

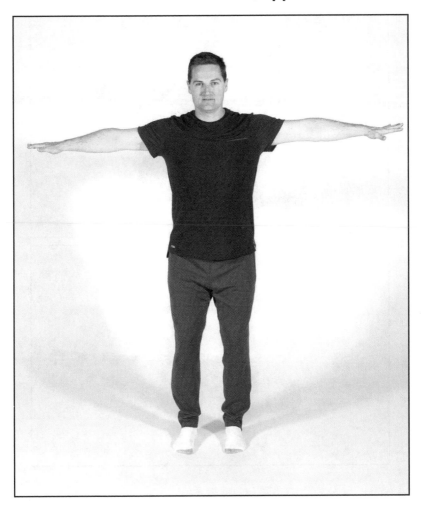

Position feet slightly wider than the hips and keep feet firmly on the floor. Holding the dumbbells to the side of the body, raise both dumbbells to approximately shoulder height. Slowly return to the starting position.

This exercise can easily be performed with a dumbbell held in each hand, standing or sitting.

47

Dead Bugs

FEEL IT HERE: stomach, legs, shoulders

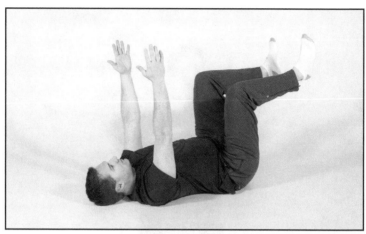

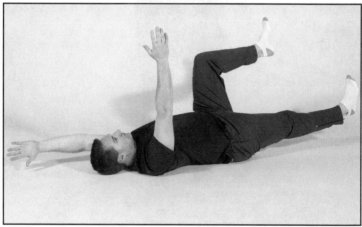

Begin by lying on your back, ideally with a towel under your lumbar spine (this is a feedback tool to help maintain a neutral spine). Bring both legs off the floor, with knees bent to 90 degrees. From this position, slowly lower one leg down while maintaining a neutral spine. Upon raising the leg back up to the starting position, alternate and lower the opposite leg. Repeat for 1–3 sets of 10–15 repetitions for each leg.

Leg Press

FEEL IT HERE: legs, hips, core

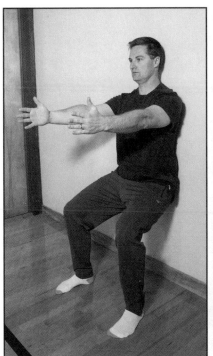 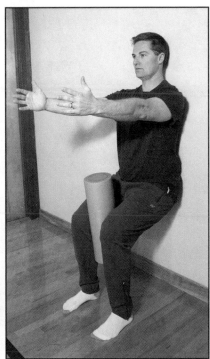

Sit down at the machine with your back fully supported, hips and knees flexed, and with your feet straight, hip to shoulder width apart. Pushing through the mid-foot and heels, extend your hips and knees until the knee is extended (keeping a slight bend to the knee so as not to lock your knee out). Slowly return to the starting position and repeat for the desired number of repetitions

Be sure to watch your breathing throughout this exercise. Keep breathing in and out; don't hold your breath, and keep your hips above the height of your knees.

Lying Triceps Elbow Extensions
FEEL IT HERE: arms, shoulders

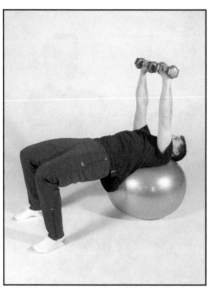 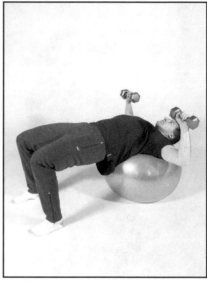

Begin by lying face up on a bench with your arms extended straight up toward the ceiling. Holding either a bar or dumbbells, slowly lower the weight toward your forehead (if using a bar) or your shoulders (if using dumbbells), keeping the upper portion of your arm perpendicular to the bench and your elbow pointing towards ceiling. Push the weight upward (making sure to keep it under control) by extending your elbows to return to the starting position.

Physioball Walk-ups

FEEL IT HERE: legs, hips, core

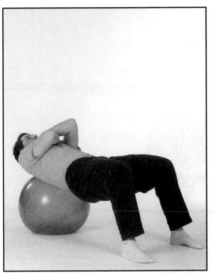

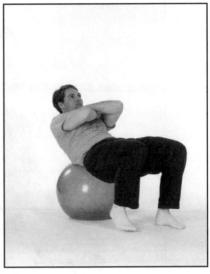

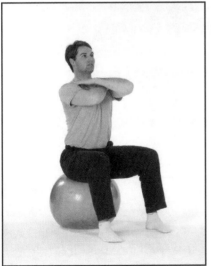

Position your hips on top of the physioball. Brace your core and walk down the ball using your full foot. Your legs, hips, and core should all be active during this exercise. Keeping your feet wider can help add stability if you feel off balance during the up or down phases.

Physioball Squat

FEEL IT HERE: legs, hips, core

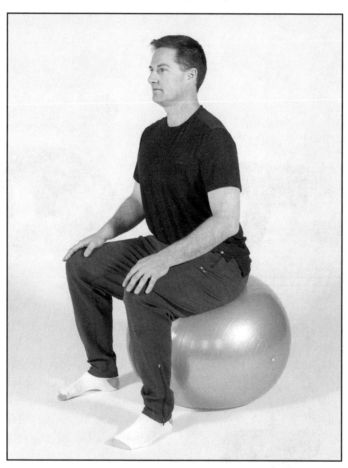

Standing over a physioball (or box), keep your arms raised and extended in front of your eyes, with your feet about shoulder width apart and toes straight ahead. Initiate the exercise by pushing your hips back with a neutral lower back, allowing your knees to bend naturally. Attempt to maintain a vertical shin as you squat down until your glutes touch the physioball, and pause for 2 seconds. Drive your heels into the ground to push yourself back up.

Push-Ups

FEEL IT HERE: chest, shoulders, core

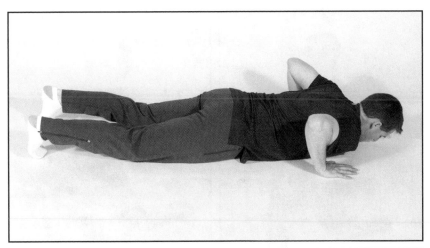

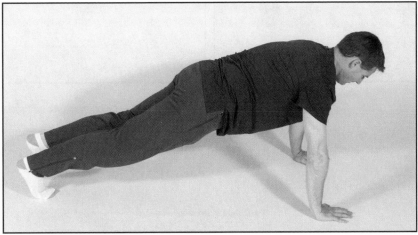

Place your hands on the floor about shoulder width apart in a plank position. Initiate the movement by pulling your shoulder blades down and back and pointing your elbows back towards your feet. Lower your chest until it touches the floor, and then press back up to the start position.

Clock Lunge

FEEL IT HERE: legs, hips, core

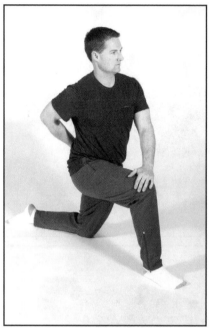 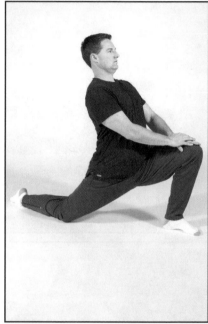

Imagine you are standing in the middle of a clock face. Lunge to various positions on the clock face. Lunging needs to be executed with proper movement at the hip and knee. Sit the hips down and back into each number on the clock face."

Reverse Lunge and Press to Single Leg Balance

FEEL IT HERE: legs, hips, core, shoulders

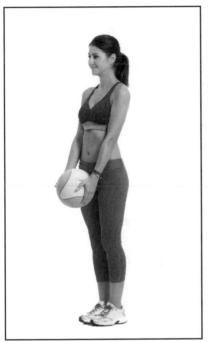 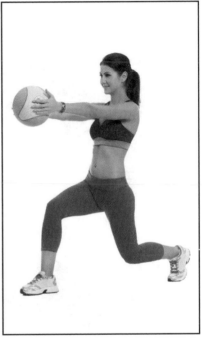

Start by standing tall with feet together holding a medicine ball or other object (i.e. dumbbell or plate) in front of the body at shoulder height. Lunge backwards by dropping one leg back so that the front leg is parallel to the floor with the knee bent at 90 degrees while pressing the medicine ball directly overhead. The back leg should be bent at the knee as well. Using the forward leg, pull your body back to the starting position and lower the medicine ball back down to shoulder level. You can progress this exercise by returning to a single leg balance position, rather than a standing upright position between repetitions. In this position, the back leg becomes flexed at the hip to approximately 90 degrees so that you are balancing/standing on the front leg.

Hip Bridge
FEEL IT HERE: hips, back

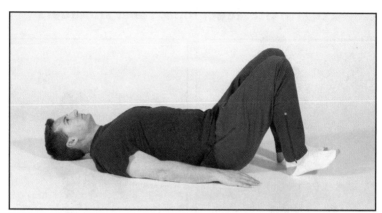

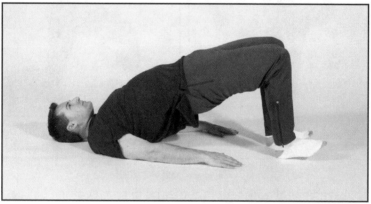

Lying supine with your knees bent and feet flat on the floor, contract your glutes and raise your hips off the floor until your body is in a straight line. Perform 1–3 sets of 10–15 repetitions.

Progress to a Single Leg Hip Bridge, then to performing the bridging action with feet on a physio/stability ball.

Single/Double Leg Deadlifts

FEEL IT HERE: legs, hips, core

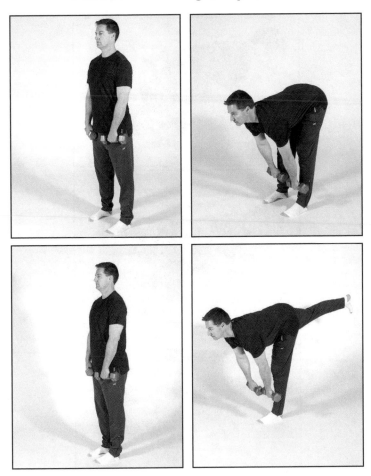

Standing up tall on one leg, place your hands on your hips and slightly bend your knees. Initiate the exercise by only moving your hips back while keeping your chest up. Initiate the exercise by kicking your balance leg back until you feel a good stretch in the hamstring of the leg on the floor. You may use an anchor point for your hands if you are having trouble balancing or if you want to emphasize stretching over balance. This variation of the movement places additional focus on the hamstrings.

Hip Circles

FEEL IT HERE: hips, core

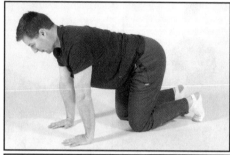

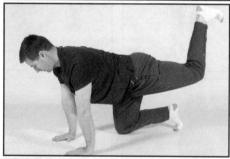

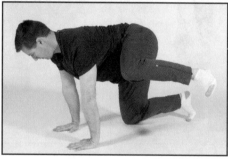

Position yourself on your hands and knees with your hands directly below your shoulders and knees directly under your hips. Your torso should be parallel to the floor with the low back flat in a neutral lumbar spine. Perform a small circle with your knee, maintaining this position. Gradually increase the size of the circle while maintaining the starting position. Perform 10–15 repetitions and then reverse the direction of the circle. Repeat on both sides for 1–3 sets.

Dumbell Row with Triceps

FEEL IT HERE: shoulders, arms

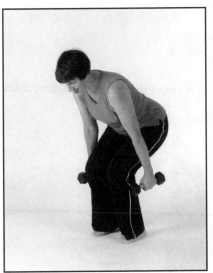

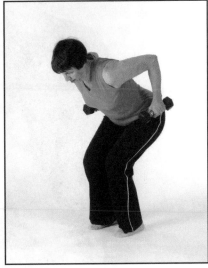

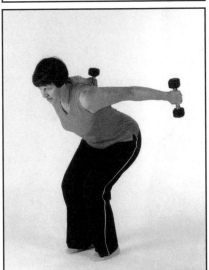

Position your feet under your hips and brace your core. Part one of this movement requires a row. Once the rowing motion has been completed, use your triceps muscle to extend your hand. Remember to position your legs with a split support base.

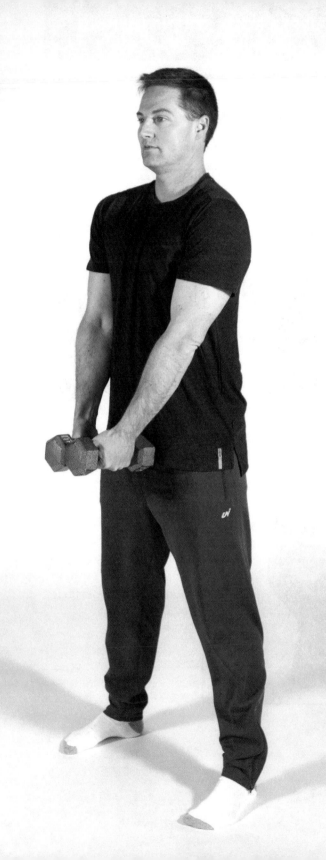

CHAPTER 5

Physical Evaluations

The following are the most up-to-date American College of Sports Medicine cardiac recovery exercise guidelines, intended as recommendations for individuals with cardiovascular disease participating in outpatient cardiac rehabilitation.

	AEROBIC	RESISTANCE	FLEXIBILITY
Frequency	Minimum of 3 days per week, preferably 5 or more days per week.	2–3 nonconsecutive days per week.	Minimum of 2–3 days per week, with daily exercise being the most effective.
Intensity	With an exercise test, 40–80 percent of exercise capacity using HRR method. Without an exercise test, use seated or standing HR + 20–30 beats, or an RPE of 12–16 on a scale of 6–20.	Perform 10–15 repetitions of each exercise without significant fatigue; RPE of 11–13 on a 6–20 scale or 40–60 percent of 1 RM.	To the point of feeling tightness or slight discomfort.
Time	20–60 minutes.	1–3 sets; 8–10 different exercises focused on major muscle groups.	15 second hold for static stretching, repeated four or more times for each exercise.
Type	Various forms may be used, including but not limited to: rower, treadmill, bike elliptical	Select equipment that is safe and comfortable for the patient to use.	Static or dynamic stretching focused on the major joints of the limbs and lower back.

AEROBIC EXERCISE

While we often classify this area of the exercise prescription as aerobic, a better term may be cardiovascular, as it encompasses all three systems of energy development. Since each of these systems play a critical role in how we perform on a daily basis, it only makes sense that an exercise program will incorporate all three.

So, what are the three systems and how do we train them? The first two systems we will briefly discuss are the ATP-PC and Glycolytic system. Each of these systems produces energy for human motion *without* the use of oxygen. However, our ability to sustain an activity is limited, as fatigue sets in quickly due to the intensity of the work being performed. The aerobic system, on the other hand, works *with* oxygen to create energy, and therefore has the ability to sustain us for very long periods of time.

Here is a simple breakdown of each system:

- ATP-PC: used for short bursts of energy up to about 15 seconds
- Glycolytic: used for longer duration, high intensity work, up to about 2:30–3 minutes
- Aerobic: used for longer duration, low to moderate intensity work lasting longer than 3 minutes

Now that we have a basic understanding of the three systems of energy production, we can begin to discuss programming for long-term cardiac health. Traditional aerobic exercise prescription was often programmed as long, slow, and distance based. While this type of program may be needed for someone who is training for a marathon, it is not a complete picture of cardiac health. The heart is a muscle, one that needs to be progressively overloaded to increase its strength and efficiency. Therefore, the programs outlined in this book will follow a systematic approach to progress you from potentially a very low level of cardiovascular efficiency to one that meets the needs of your activities of daily living and beyond. All programs will follow the guidelines outlined in previous sections in accordance with the American College of Sports Medicine.

These different degrees of progressive difficulty will be referred to as levels. Level 1 is designed to build overall tolerance to exercise, working at a constant intensity with the duration of the session gradually increasing from week to week. While the program starts off at a frequency of three days per week, you may increase this as tolerated. You will be working at an intensity that is classified as fairly light to somewhat hard.

LEVEL 1			
	WEEK 1	**WEEK 2**	**WEEK 3**
DAY 1	20 minutes continuous exercise at 40–50 percent of HRR or an RPE of 11–13	20–25 minutes continuous exercise at 40–50 percent of HRR or an RPE of 11–13	25–30 minutes continuous exercise at 40 – 50 percent of HRR or an RPE of 11–13
DAY 2	Recovery day	Recovery day	Recovery day
DAY 3	20 minutes continuous exercise at 40–50 percent of HRR or an RPE of 11–13	20–25 minutes continuous exercise at 40–50 percent of HRR or an RPE of 11–13	25–30 minutes continuous exercise at 40–50 percent of HRR or an RPE of 11–13
DAY 4	Recovery day	Recovery day	Recovery day
DAY 5	20 minutes continuous exercise at 40–50 percent of HRR or an RPE of 11–13	20–25 minutes continuous exercise at 40–50 percent of HRR or an RPE of 11–13	25–30 minutes continuous exercise at 40–50 percent of HRR or an RPE of 11–13

Programming in Level 2 becomes more progressive with the introduction of interval training. The goal is to increase the frequency and overall session intensity while continuing to progress the duration of the session. You will also see the inclusion of shorter duration sessions at a higher intensity than previously programmed.

	WEEK 1	WEEK 2	WEEK 3
LEVEL 2			
DAY 1	30 minutes continuous exercise at 50–60 percent of HRR or an RPE of 12–14	30–35 minutes continuous exercise at 50–60 percent of HRR or an RPE of 12–14	30–35 minutes continuous exercise at 50–60 percent of HRR or an RPE of 12–14
DAY 2	Interval Training Work: 1 minute at 60–65 percent of HRR Recovery: 3 minutes at a comfortable pace Repeat: 5–6 times	Interval Training Work: 2 minutes at 60–65 percent of HRR Recovery: 2 minutes at a comfortable pace Repeat: 5–6 times	Interval Training Work: 1 minute at 65–70 percent of HRR Recovery: 3 minutes at a comfortable pace Repeat: 5–6 times
DAY 3	30 minutes continuous exercise at 50–60 percent of HRR or an RPE of 12–14	30–35 minutes continuous exercise at 50–60 percent of HRR or an RPE of 12–14	25–30 minutes continuous exercise at 50–60 percent of HRR or an RPE of 12–14
DAY 4	Recovery day	Recovery day	Recovery day
DAY 5	20–30 minutes continuous exercise at 55–65 percent of HRR or an RPE of 13–15	20–30 minutes continuous exercise at 55–65 percent of HRR or an RPE of 13–15	25–30 minutes continuous exercise at 55–65 percent of HRR or an RPE of 13–15

Level 3 continues to progress the frequency, intensity, and time of each session. We also begin to increase the intensity of the interval training sessions, either by increasing the rate (percentage intensity or RPE) at which the work is performed or by decreasing the amount of recovery time.

LEVEL 3		
	WEEK 1	**WEEK 2**	**WEEK 3**
DAY 1	30 minutes continuous exercise at 55–65 percent of HRR or an RPE of 13–15	30–35 minutes continuous exercise at 55–65 percent of HRR or an RPE of 13–15	Interval Training Work: 3 minutes @ 70–75 percent of HRR Recovery: 1 minutes at a comfortable pace Repeat: 5–6 times
DAY 2	Interval Training Work: 1 minute @ 70–75 percent of HRR Recovery: 2 minutes at a comfortable pace Repeat: 5–6 times	Interval Training Work: 2 minutes @ 70–75 percent of HRR Recovery: 2 minutes at a comfortable pace Repeat: 5–6 times	25–30 minutes continuous exercise at 65–70 percent of HRR or an RPE of 13–15
DAY 3	30 minutes continuous exercise at 55–65 percent of HRR or an RPE of 13–15	30–35 minutes continuous exercise at 55–65 percent of HRR or an RPE of 13–15	Interval Training Work: 3 minutes @ 70–75 percent of HRR Recovery: 1 minutes at a comfortable pace Repeat: 5–6 times
DAY 4	Interval Training Work: 1 minute @ 70–75 percent of HRR Recovery: 2 minutes at a comfortable pace Repeat: 5–6 times	Interval Training Work: 2 minutes @ 70–75 percent of HRR Recovery: 1 minutes at a comfortable pace Repeat: 5–6 times	25–30 minutes continuous exercise at 65–70 percent of HRR or an RPE of 13–15

DAY 5	20–30 minutes continuous exercise at 65–70 percent of HRR or an RPE of 13–15	20–30 minutes continuous exercise at 65–70 percent of HRR or an RPE of 13–15	Interval Training Work: 3 minutes @ 70–75 percent of HRR Recovery: 1 minutes at a comfortable pace Repeat: 5–6 times

RESISTANCE TRAINING

Resistance training is an important component to any fitness program. This becomes even more evident when cardiac recovery is the focus. Not only does resistance training provide a stimulus to the cardiovascular system, it also increases our economy of movement, meaning that we become more efficient with our normal daily tasks or ADLs. Think about this way: if we increase our levels of muscular fitness (i.e. strength and endurance), everything we do becomes easier and thereby places less stress of the heart.

TYPES OF MOVEMENTS

When designing a resistance training program for cardiac recovery and health, exercises should include compound, multi-joint movements that work the major muscle groups of the body. These include exercises like squats, lunges, step-ups, upper body pushing and pulling, just to name few. We will also include some single joint, isolation exercises as deemed appropriate. This is not only a time-efficient way to train, but also places the most demand and stimulus on the body creating a better dose response per workout. These exercises are also considered more functional in nature and have a better carry over to everyday life.

We will employ many of the same principles seen in the previous section for what is traditionally called aerobic fitness. The program will be progressive, adding both volume and intensity over the course of several weeks. This will allow for sufficient time to adapt to the new training stimulus. Unlike cardiovascular training, the frequency will be much less, based on the fact that more recovery is needed between sessions to allow the muscles involved to repair and regenerate, thereby getting stronger. Too much volume or frequency in the beginning will not allow you to have sufficient recovery between sessions.

You'll also find a programmed progression from variable resistance equipment (as found in most health clubs and fitness centers) to body weight and free weight exercises, and finally to suspension style exercises performed on a TRX Suspension System or similar equipment. This progression model helps to continuously overload the muscular system and provide a new training stimulus as you progress through the program. As you become familiar with the exercises, you may begin to systematically swap out exercises for other, biomechanically similar ones.

PROGRAM VARIABLES	LEVEL 1	LEVEL 2	LEVEL 3
DURATION	2–4 weeks	2–4 weeks	2–4 weeks
SETS PER EXERCISE	1–3	≥ 3	≥ 3
REPS PER SET	12–15	10–12	6–12
REST BETWEEN SETS	30 seconds	30–60 seconds	30–90 seconds
LOAD/INTENSITY (% 1 RM)	40–60%	60–70%	70–80%

PRIMARY EXERCISE PROGRESSIONS BASED ON MOVEMENT PATTERN				
MOVEMENT PATTERN	PROGRESSION 1	PROGRESSION 2	PROGRESSION 3	PROGRESSION 4
Bilateral Lower Body Pattern	Leg Press	Wall Sit/Ball Squat	Goblet Squat	Back Squat
Unilateral Lower Body Pattern	Clock Lunge	Forward or Reverse Lunge	Lateral Lunge	Multiplanar Lunge
Hip Extension/ Hinge	Hip/Glute Bridge	Deadlift	Single Leg Deadlift	Kettlebell Swing
Horizontal Push/Press	Machine Chest Press	Push Up (and variations)	Barbell Bench Press	Dumbbell Chest Press
Horizontal Pull	Dumbbell Double Arm Row	Dumbbell Row Chest Supported	Dumbbell Single Arm Row	Bent Over Row
Vertical Pull	Lateral Pulldown	Assisted Chin Up	Chin Up	Pull Ups
Vertical Push/ Press	Machine Shoulder Press	Dumbbell Overhead Press	Dumbbell Overhead Press	Bicep Curl to Press

MOVEMENT PATTERN	PROGRESSION 1	PROGRESSION 2	PROGRESSION 3
Quads	Leg Extension	Leg Extension (Single Leg)	
Hamstrings	Lying Leg Curls	Seated Leg Curls	Physioball Leg Curls
Shoulders	Front Raise	Lateral Raise	Posterior Raise
Biceps	Machine Curls	Dumbbell Curls	
Triceps	Triceps Pushdown	Triceps Kickbacks	Lying Triceps Elbow Extensions

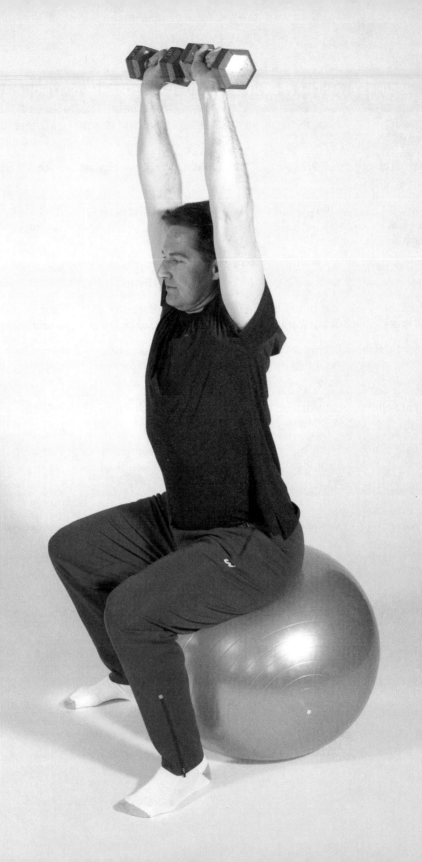

The Strong Heart Fitness Program

PROGRAMS

Introductory

- Complete Functional and Physical Assessments

Begin Cardiac Recovery: Pick your primary focus

- Start Workout A

OR

- Start Workout B

OR

- Start Workout C

Intermediate

- Start Workout A

OR

- Start Workout B

OR

- Start Workout C

Advanced

- Start Workout A

OR

- Start Workout B

OR

- Start Workout C

Integrated Program: Full Body Workouts

- Start progression Workout A: Introductory
- Start progression Workout B: Intermediate
- Start progression Workout C: Advanced

ASSESSMENTS

INITIAL EVALUATION DATE (WEEK I)

FUNCTIONAL ASSESSMENT	COMPLETE (YES/NO)	DISCOMFORT (YES/NO)	NOTE DIFFICULTY
Stair Walking			
Single Leg Balancing			
Overhead Squat			
Back Extension			
Over/Under: Back Scratch			
Clock Lunge			

PHYSICAL FITNESS ASSESSMENT	GOAL	INITIAL	MID-POINT	SUM-MARY
Cooper Test (run as far as possible in 12 minutes)				
Push-ups				
Pull-up/Flex-arm Hang				
Wall Sits				

MID-POINT EVALUATION DATE (WEEK 6)

FUNCTIONAL ASSESSMENT	COMPLETE (YES/NO)	DISCOMFORT (YES/NO)	NOTE DIFFICULTY
Stair Walking			
Single Leg Balancing			
Overhead Squat			
Back Extension			
Over/Under: Back Scratch			
Clock Lunge			

PHYSICAL FITNESS ASSESSMENT	GOAL	INITIAL	MID-POINT	SUMMARY
Cooper Test (run as far as possible in 12 minutes)				
Push-ups				
Pull-up/Flex-arm Hang				
Wall Sits				

SUMMARY EVALUATION DATE (WEEK 12)

FUNCTIONAL ASSESSMENT	COMPLETE (YES/NO)	DISCOMFORT (YES/NO)	NOTE DIFFICULTY
Stair Walking			
Single Leg Balancing			
Overhead Squat			
Back Extension			
Over/Under: Back Scratch			
Clock Lunge			

PHYSICAL FITNESS ASSESSMENT	GOAL	INITIAL	MID-POINT	SUM-MARY
Cooper Test (run as far as possible in 12 minutes)				
Push-ups				
Pull-up/Flex-arm Hang				
Wall Sits				

Beginner Workouts

BEGINNER (LEVEL 1)
Reps: 12–15 • **Sets:** 1–3 • **Rate of Perceived Exertion:** 3/10

EXERCISE	PAGE #	EQUIPMENT
Leg Press		Leg Press Machine
Dead Bugs		
Physioball Walk-ups		Physioball
Upright Row with Band		Band(s)
Dumbbell Chest Press		Dumbbell(s)
Lateral Raise		Dumbbell(s)
Bicep Curls		Dumbbell(s)
Dumbbell Row with Triceps Extension		Dumbbell(s)

BEGINNER (LEVEL 2)
Reps: 12–15 • **Sets:** 1–3 • **Rate of Perceived Exertion:** 3/10

EXERCISE	PAGE #	EQUIPMENT
Leg Press		Leg Press Machine
Dead Bugs		
Hip Bridge		
Dumbbell Double Arm Row		Dumbbell(s)
Dumbbell Chest Press		Dumbbell(s)
Saws		
Bicep Curls		Dumbbell(s)
Hip Circles		

BEGINNER (LEVEL 3)

Reps: 12–15 • **Sets:** 1–3 • **Rate of Perceived Exertion:** 3/10

EXERCISE	PAGE #	EQUIPMENT
Physioball Squat		Physioball
Stationary Lunge/ Split Squat		
Push-Ups		
Band Pull-Aparts		Band(s)
Bicep Curls		Dumbbell(s)
Lying Triceps Elbow Extensions		Dumbbell(s)

Intermediate Workouts

INTERMEDIATE (LEVEL 1)

Reps: 10–12 • **Sets:** 3 • **Rate of Perceived Exertion:** 5/10

EXERCISE	PAGE #	EQUIPMENT
Clock Lunge		
Physioball Walk-ups		Physioball
Dumbbell Chest Press		Dumbbell(s)
Dumbbell Double Arm Row		Dumbbell(s)
Bicep Curl to Shoulder Press		Dumbbell(s)
Dumbbell Row with Triceps Extension		Dumbbell(s)

INTERMEDIATE (LEVEL 2)

Reps: 10–12 • **Sets:** 3 • **Rate of Perceived Exertion:** 5/10

EXERCISE	PAGE #	EQUIPMENT
Goblet Squat		Kettlebell/Dumbbell
Glute Bridge		
Upright Row with Band		Band(s)
Dumbbell Chest Press		Dumbbell(s)
Band Pull-Aparts		Band(s)
Bicep Curls		Dumbbell(s)
Hip Circles		

INTERMEDIATE (LEVEL 3)

Reps: 10–12 • **Sets:** 3 • **Rate of Perceived Exertion:** 5/10

EXERCISE	PAGE #	EQUIPMENT
Body Weight Squat		
Glute Bridge		
Dumbbell Single Arm Row		Dumbbell(s)
Dumbbell Chest Press		Dumbbell(s)
Dumbbell Overhead Press		Dumbbell(s)
Bicep Curls		Dumbbell(s)
Lying Triceps Elbow Extensions		Dumbbell(s)

Advanced Workouts

ADVANCED (LEVEL 1)

Reps: 6–10 • **Sets:** 3–4 • **Rate of Perceived Exertion:** 7/10

EXERCISE	PAGE #	EQUIPMENT
Spiderman		
Deadlift		Barbell
Dumbbell Chest Press		Dumbbell(s)
Dumbbell Row		Dumbbell(s)
Bicep Curl to Shoulder Press		Dumbbell(s)
Lying Triceps Elbow Extensions		Dumbbell(s)

ADVANCED (LEVEL 2)

Reps: 6–10 • **Sets:** 3 • **Rate of Perceived Exertion:** 7/10

EXERCISE	PAGE #	EQUIPMENT
Goblet Squat to Shoulder Press		Kettlebell/Dumbbell
Single Leg Deadlift		Barbell
Draw the Sword		Band(s)
Dumbbell Chest Press		Dumbbell(s)
Dumbbell Overhead Press		Dumbbell(s)
Bicep Curls		Dumbbell(s)
Hip Circles		

ADVANCED (LEVEL 3)

Reps: 6–10 • **Sets:** 3 • **Rate of Perceived Exertion:** 7/10

EXERCISE	PAGE #	EQUIPMENT
Body Weight Squat		
Glute Bridge		
Dumbbell Single Arm Row		Dumbbell(s)
Incline Dumbbell Chest Press		Dumbbell(s)
Dumbbell Overhead Press		Dumbbells
Bicep Curls		Dumbbell(s)
Triceps Pushdowns		Barbell

Integrated Workouts

INTEGRATED CARDIAC RECOVERY WORKOUTS (LEVEL 1)

Reps: 6–12 • **Sets:** 3–4 • **Rate of Perceived Exertion:** 7/10

EXERCISE	PAGE #	EQUIPMENT
Superset: Goblet Squat and Dumbbell Chest Press		Kettlebell/Dumbbell(s)
Superset: Alternate Lunges and Dumbbell Rows		Dumbbell(s)
Superset: Physioball Walk-ups and Bicep Curl to Press		Physioball, Dumbbell(s)

INTEGRATED CARDIAC RECOVERY WORKOUTS (LEVEL 2)

Reps: 6–12 • **Sets:** 3–4 • **Rate of Perceived Exertion:** 7/10

EXERCISE	PAGE #	EQUIPMENT
Clock Lunge		
Superset: Upright Rows (with Band) and Push-Ups		Band(s)
Superset: Dumbbell Chest Press and Dumbbell Single Arm Row		Dumbbell(s)
Band Pull-Aparts		Band(s)
Superset: Lying Triceps Elbow Extensions and Bicep Curls		Dumbbell(s)

INTEGRATED CARDIAC RECOVERY WORKOUTS (LEVEL 3)

Reps: 6–12 • **Sets:** 3–4 • **Rate of Perceived Exertion:** 7/10

EXERCISE	PAGE #	EQUIPMENT
Multiplanar Lunge Complex: Forward, Reverse, and Lateral		
Dumbbell Squat		Dumbbell(s)
Single Leg Deadlift		Dumbbell(s)
Dumbbell Rows		Dumbbell(s)
Dumbbell Chest Press		Dumbbell(s)
Bicep Curl to Shoulder Press		Dumbbell(s)

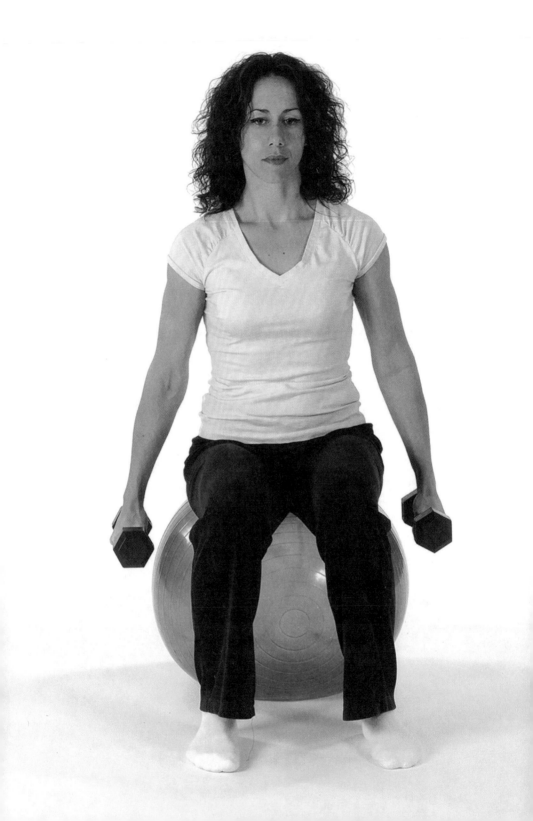

APPENDIX A:
COMMONLY USED CARDIAC
TERMINOLOGY

Acute Care: Secondary health care in which a patient receives active short-term treatment for injury or illness, or during recovery from surgery.

Blood Pressure: Blood pressure can be broken down into two types—systolic and diastolic. Systolic is the pressure created when the heart exerts force, and diastolic is the pressure created upon the return of blood to the heart. Normal blood pressure is defined as 120/80, with the systolic figure on top, and diastolic figure on the bottom.

Body Mass Index: A measurement of height and weight.

Cardiorespiratory System: An umbrella term which includes the heart, lungs, and vessels, which work together to deliver oxygen to working muscles.

Edema: swelling caused by excess fluid trapped in the body's tissues.

Heart Rate Reserve: The difference between resting heart rate and maximum heart rate, used to determine appropriate exercise heart rates.

Hypertension: Also known as high blood pressure, in which the force of the blood against the artery walls is high enough that it could eventually cause health problems such as heart disease.

Hypotension: Low blood pressure; the opposite of hypertension.

Ischemia: A lack of oxygen.

Orthostatic Hypotension: A form of low blood pressure that occurs when standing up from sitting/lying down, which can make you feel dizzy and lightheaded.

Outpatient Care: Medical care provided on an outpatient basis, including diagnosis, observation, consultation, treatment, intervention, and rehabilitation services.

Pulse Rate: The number of heart beats per minute; the average resting rate for an adult is 60-80 BPM (beats per minute).

Resting Heart Rate: The number of times the heart beats per minute while resting; can be used as an indicator of physical fitness.

Stress Test: A test of cardiovascular strength done by monitoring heart rate during increasingly strenuous exercise.

Sub-Acute: A medical condition that falls between sudden onset (acute) and a condition with an indefinite duration (chronic).

Syncope: Partial or complete loss of consciousness caused by a sudden drop in blood pressure.

Target Heart Rate Zone: A personalized pulse rate to be maintained during exercise to reach optimal cardiovascular function; usually 60-85% of the maximum heart rate.

Working Rate: see *Target Heart Rate Zone*

APPENDIX B:
GLOSSARY OF EXERCISE TERMINOLOGY

Aerobic: Exercise that improves the efficiency of the cardiovascular system in obtaining oxygen from breathing.

Anaerobic: Short duration, high intensity exercise that is not intended to improve the cardiovascular system's ability to obtain oxygen from breathing.

Closed Chain Exercise: Exercises performed in which the hand or foot is in a fixed position and does not move.

Compound Movement: Exercises that engage multiple joints to train entire muscle groups.

Load: The amount of weight one lifts in relation to repetitions.

Open Chain Exercise: Exercises performed in which the hand or foot is free to move.

Rate of Perceived Exertion (RPE): A scale used to measure the perceived intensity of an exercise.

Rate of Recovery: The decrease in the heart rate from peak exercise until one minute after exercise ends.

Repetition (Rep): One complete motion of an exercise.

Set: A group of consecutive repetitions.

Talk-test: A test used to measure the intensity of an exercise; during moderate intensity you can talk, and during vigorous intensity you should not be able to say more than a few words without needing to take a breath.

Volume: The amount of work one does while exercising, such as the number of reps performed in one session.

Work Rest Ration (W/R): The amount of work (exercise) done in a session compared to the amount of rest.

CARDIAC QUICK-FIXES AND "LIFE-HACKS"

CARDIAC RECOVERY QUICK REFERENCE GUIDES

Try some of these quick-and-easy "mini-workouts" when on-the-go or at your desk for an on-demand cardiac fix!

Quick Reference Desk #1: The 3-Minute Home Solution

- Physioball Squats (15 seconds)
- Stair Stepping (20 seconds)
- Spiderman (15 seconds)
- Take your pulse rate for 10 seconds and multiply the result by 6. Try to keep your heart rate at 30 above resting pulse.

Repeat if you are able. Work up to 3 rounds.

CARDIAC RECOVERY "LIFE-HACKS"

Heart disease and its related risk factors are generally preventable. While you cannot control your family health history, you *can* control the daily habits that trigger a cardiac event.

Stress is a major contributor to low-level inflammation. Inflammation, when unmanaged over long periods of time, is detrimental to one's overall health. Low levels of cortisol are released during periods of stress, causing systemic inflammation. Managing daily stressors is key to not only an optimally functioning cardiovascular system but the prevention of other diseases where inflammation is a contribution factor. These include cancer, diabetes, arterial diseases and rheumatic conditions.

5 Cardiac "Life-Hacks" for the Office

- Take the stairs instead of the elevator
- Park further away from your building

- Grab a buddy for an afternoon partner walk
- Participate in your employer-sponsored cholesterol screenings
- Host a heart-healthy lecture at your place of employment with a local healthcare system

5 Cardiac "Life-Hacks" for the Home

- Take the stairs when possible
- Understand your pulse rate, taking it morning, noon and night
- Use alternative seasonings to salt
- Practice deep breathing daily and keep a "To-Do" list for managing time
- Eat breakfast everyday

5 Cardiac "Life-Hacks" for the Caregivers

- Work on balance and mobility, and practice transferring weight from side to side
- Daily stretching can alleviate strain, making movement less strenuous
- When using a physioball, the ball should be slightly above the height of the knee to ensure proper height. When sitting, the hips should be slightly above the knees.
- During daily walks, use the Talk Test. If your sentences are broken, that tells you the 'aerobic' threshold is being reached.
- Target the upper back, hips and legs with strengthening exercises

RECOMMENDED GYM EQUIPMENT

EXERCISE NAME	RECOMMENDED EQUIPMENT
Band Pull Apart	Reverse Cable Flyes
Dumbbell Chest Press	Machine Chest Press
Spiderman	Yoga/Pilates/Stretching Rack
Dumbbell Rows	Upright Row
Dumbbell Overhead Press	Machine Shoulder Press
Dumbbell Squat	—
Bicep Curl to Shoulder Press	Sitting Biceps Curl and Machine Shoulder Press
Bicep Curls	Sitting Biceps Curl
Body Weight Squat	—
Dumbbell Deadlifts	Use Barbell in Gym
Dumbbell Double Arm Row	Upright Row
Dumbbell Single Arm Row	Upright Row or Single Arm Cable Pull
Saws	Upright Row or Cable Pull
Glute Bridge	Hip Lift on Physioball
Goblet Squat	Use Kettlebell or Medicine Ball in Gym
Incline Dumbbell Chest Press	Machine Incline Press
Upright Row with Band	Upright Row Machine
Draw the Sword	Reverse Cable Flyes
Lateral Raise	Use Lateral Cable Raise
Dead Bugs	Plank
Leg Press	Use Horizontal Leg Press in Gym
Lying Triceps Elbow Extensions	Cable or Machine Triceps Pressdown
Physioball Walk-ups	Step Ups
Physioball Squat	—
Push-Ups	Machine Chest Press
Clock Lunge	Hip Adduction/Abduction Machine
Reverse Lunge and Press to Single Leg Balance	Walking Lunge and Machine Shoulder Press
Hip Bridge	—
Single/Double Leg Deadlifts	Machine Sitting Hamstring Leg Curl
Hip Circles	Hip Adduction/Abduction Machine
Dumbbell Row with Triceps	Upright Rows and Machine or Cable Pressdowns

RESOURCES

CONTINUING CARE:
COMMUNITY-BASED RESOURCES

Community-based cardiac health programs have come a long way in the last 30 years. Long gone are days of having someone walk on the treadmill for 45 minutes.

While there are still sections of the population that need that sort of basic, steady state exercise (such as those recently discharged from medical care), for those of you reading this book with no significant cardiac risk factors, new training approaches which integrate advancements like kettlebells, TRX suspension, spinning and interval training provide non-traditional resources for those looking to see more reliable results. Remember: it's not the tool or type of training program you use that matters; it is the application of proven principles of exercise program design (including work/rest ratios) that makes the difference and sees results.

As we've mentioned, getting heart-healthy means making a commitment to certain lifestyle and behavior changes. Once a patient becomes a "regular" person—transitioning from hospital-based care to self-care—they need to also transition into a comprehensive, cardiac-focused program. Luckily, health care institutions will often be able to provide you with the names of local fitness and health facilities that already offer basic post-rehabilitative programs. These will commonly go by titles like "Heart Success" or "Cardiac Fit" programs. This basic approach should also feature an initial evaluation by an exercise specialist, which must include a medical history, sub-max bike or treadmill test, blood pressure and machine orientation.

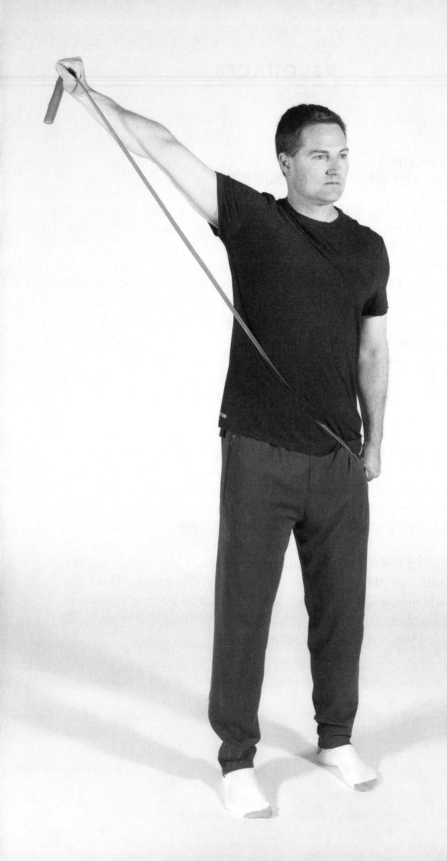

ABOUT THE AUTHORS

William Smith, MS, NSCA-CSCS, MEPD

Will currently works for a nationally recognized healthcare system in the New York metropolitan area providing health and wellness services to the community. His interest is in special populations and how healthcare providers and fitness professionals can work more closely together.

Will completed his B.S. in exercise science followed by an MS at St. John's University where he was the Assistant Director of Strength and Conditioning. Will has been featured on NBC, Canyon Ranch, World Spinning Conference and in *Homecare Magazine*.

Chris Volgraf, CSCS, cEP, FRCms, TPI-Level 2

Chris completed his B.S. in exercise science at Temple University, where he specialized in exercise testing and prescription. During his years in the profession he has been featured in Philadelphia local news, ABC national news and *Opera Magazine*.

Chris is currently the owner and Head Strength & Conditioning Coach of Clutch Performance and Fitness, a premier sports performance and fitness training company in the Philadelphia/Princeton area. Chris has worked with professional, amateur, collegiate and high school athletes for the past 13 years. Chris is also a founding employee of the Princeton Longevity Center in Princeton, NJ, where he served as the Director of Fitness and the Senior Exercise Physiologist for 14 years.

Keith Burns, MS, CSCS

Keith graduated in 2008 with a Master of Science in Human Movement with a concentration in Corrective Exercise from Arizona School of Health Sciences, A.T. Still University.

Keith has served in almost every capacity of the exercise science field at both the collegiate and professional level, working primarily as a strength and conditioning coach. His professional experiences also includes working with several baseball organizations as a strength and conditioning coach, including the Chicago White Sox, Philadelphia Phillies, and Detroit Tigers. Keith has also worked for two national sports performance franchises, Velocity Sports Performance and the Parisi Speed School. Keith currently works as a tenured track Instructor of Exercise Science at Raritan Valley Community College.

ALSO IN THIS SERIES

getfitnow

GOT QUESTIONS?
NEED ANSWERS?
GO TO:
GETFITNOW.COM

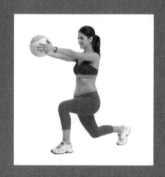 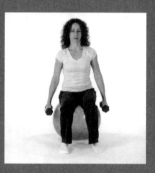 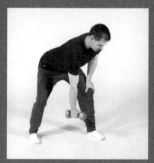

IT'S FITNESS 24/7

Videos, Workouts, Nutrition,
Recipes, Community Tips, and more!